ROLE OF NEUTROPHILS IN DISEASE PATHOGENESIS

Edited by **Maitham Abbas Khajah**

Role of Neutrophils in Disease Pathogenesis
http://dx.doi.org/10.5772/65581
Edited by Maitham Abbas Khajah

Contributors

MMaximinaBertha Moreno-Altamirano, Christian Eduardo Cruz-Gómez, Lluvia E López-Luis, Elaine Cruz Rosas, Luana Correa, Maria Das Graças Henriques, Adriana Bonomo, Suelen Perobelli, Triciana Gonçalves-Silva, Eileen Uribe-Querol, Carlos Rosales, Maria Rapala-Kozik, Marcin Zawrotniak, Andrzej Kozik, Massimo Conese, Stefano Castellani, Susanna D'Oria, Sante Di Gioia, Pasqualina Montemurro, Zsolt Balogh, Gabrielle Briggs

Published by InTech
Janeza Trdine 9, 51000 Rijeka, Croatia

Publishing Process Manager Romina Rovan
Technical Editor SPi Global
Cover InTech Design team

First published May, 2017
Printed in Croatia
Legal deposit, Croatia: National and University Library in Zagreb

Additional hard copies can be obtained from orders@intechopen.com

Role of Neutrophils in Disease Pathogenesis, Edited by Maitham Abbas Khajah
p. cm.
Print ISBN 978-953-51-3195-3
Online ISBN 978-953-51-3196-0

For EU product safety concerns:
IN TECH d.o.o., Prolaz Marije Krucifikse Kozulić 3, 51000 Rijeka, Croatia,
info@intechopen.com or visit our website at intechopen.com.

Meet the editor

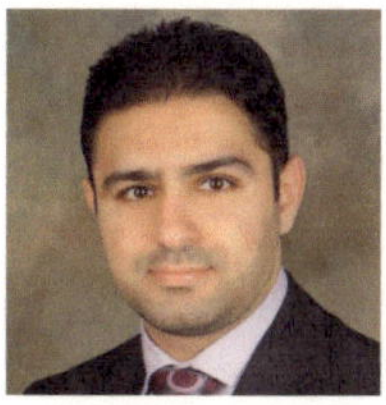

Dr. Maitham A. Khajah has completed his B Pharm degree from Faculty of Pharmacy, Kuwait University, in 2003 and obtained his PhD degree in December 2009 from the University of Calgary, Canada (Gastrointestinal Science and Immunology). He is currently an assistant professor in Kuwait University, Faculty of Pharmacy, Department of Pharmacology and Therapeutics since January 2010. His research interest is to study new molecular targets for the treatment of inflammatory bowel disease (IBD) and the mechanisms responsible for immune cell chemotaxis. He cosupervised many students for the MSc Molecular Biology Program, College of Graduate Studies, Kuwait University. Since he joined Kuwait University in 2010, he got various grants as PI and Co-I. He was awarded the Best Young Researcher Award by Kuwait University, Research Sector, for the Year 2013–2014. He was a member in the organizing committee for three conferences organized by Kuwait University, Faculty of Pharmacy, as cochair and a member in the scientific committee (the 3rd, 4th, and 5th Kuwait International Pharmacy Conference).

Contents

Preface

Neutrophils are the most abundant circulating white blood cells, which are considered the first line of innate immune response against various insults and an important link to activate the adaptive immune response when needed. They play an important role in the pathogenesis of various infectious and noninfectious diseases. Recent discovery regarding the formation of weblike structures in the extracellular space called neutrophil extracellular traps (NETs) provided better understanding of their role in various disease conditions and for their role as an important future therapeutic target.

This book *Role of Neutrophils in Disease Pathogenesis* provides the most recent evidence regarding the role of neutrophil in various diseases of infectious and noninfectious origin. The first section of this book [Section 1: Neutrophil Extracellular Traps (NETs)] focuses on the role of NETs in various diseases. Chapter 1 (Neutrophil Extracellular Traps in Infectious Human Diseases) provides a general background information regarding the mechanisms and various triggers of NET formation. The role of NETs in selected infectious and noninfectious diseases is also discussed. Chapter 2 (Beneficial and Deleterious Effects of Neutrophil Extracellular Traps on Infection) mainly focuses on providing recent evidence for the role of NETs in various infectious diseases. The various cells producing NETs, their role in the immune response, and the pros and cons of NETs are also discussed in this chapter. Chapter 3 (The Role of Neutrophil Extracellular Traps in Postinjury Inflammation) focuses on the role of NET-derived neutrophils in the pathological mechanisms leading to postinjury inflammation and secondary tissue injury. The clinical relevance of NETs in postinjury complications and the therapeutic potential of NET inhibition/clearance are also discussed at the end of this chapter.

In the second section of the book (Section 2: Neutrophil Role in Disease Pathogenesis), the role of neutrophils in the pathogenesis of selected disease conditions is discussed. Chapter 4 (Neutrophil Role in Periodontal Disease) focuses on the role of neutrophils in the pathogenesis of periodontal diseases, which leads to tooth loss or increases the risk of developing various systemic diseases in severe cases. Novel therapeutic approaches for periodontitis are also discussed at the end of this chapter. Chapter 5 (Neutrophils in Rheumatoid Arthritis: A Target for Discovering New Therapies Based on Natural Products) discusses the role of neutrophil in the initiation and progression of rheumatoid arthritis (RA). Current pharmacological treatments with their drawbacks and various substances derived from natural products as putative antirheumatic therapies are also discussed at the end of this chapter. Chapter 6 (Role of Neutrophils in Cystic Fibrosis Lung Disease) highlights the important role of neutrophils in the pathogenesis of cystic fibrosis (CF) and the utility of using these cells as a noninvasive biomarker and a readout to determine the efficacy of etiological therapies in CF.

The last section of this chapter (Section 3: Immunosuppressive Properties of Neutrophils) highlights the immunosuppressive properties of neutrophils. Chapter 7 (Neutrophil Plasticity: The Regulatory Interface in Various Pathological Conditions) focuses on an important yet less-recognized role for neutrophils in *reducing* the inflammatory responses either by direct interaction with other cells or secretion of factors to modulate the activity of the inflammatory response. More emphasis is given to their role in graft versus host disease (GVHD), which is the main limitation of allogeneic hematopoietic stem cell transplantation.

We hope that the recent evidence described in this book provides a better understanding of the role of these immune cells in various disease conditions and forms the basis for future research activities aiming to provide better therapeutic approaches to treat various disease conditions.

Dr. Maitham A. Khajah, B Pharm, PhD
Assistant Professor
Department of Pharmacology & Therapeutics
Faculty of Pharmacy, Kuwait University, Kuwait

Section 1

Neutrophil Extracellular Traps (NETs)

Chapter 1

Neutrophil Extracellular Traps in Infectious Human Diseases

Marcin Zawrotniak, Andrzej Kozik and
Maria Rapala-Kozik

Additional information is available at the end of the chapter

http://dx.doi.org/10.5772/intechopen.68443

Abstract

Neutrophils, as the main cells of the first line of host defense against microbial pathogens, are responsible for pathogen recognition, inhibition of pathogen spreading into the host tissue, and finally, killing the invader cells. Neutrophils carry out these functions via numerous mechanisms, including a relatively recently described activity based on a release of neutrophil extracellular traps (NETs), a process called netosis. NETs are structures composed of DNA backbone, decorated with antimicrobial factors, derived from neutrophil granules. The structure of NETs and their enzymatic and microbicidal inclusions enable efficient trapping and killing of microorganisms within the neutrophil extracellular space. However, the efficiency of NETs depends on neutrophil ability to recognize pathogen signals and to trigger rapid responses. In this chapter, we focus on possible pathways involved in the release of NETs and summarize the current knowledge on triggers of this process during bacterial, fungal, protozoan, and viral infections. We also consider the mechanisms used by microorganisms to evade NET-killing activity and analyze the harmful potential of NETs against the host cells and the contribution of NETs to noninfectious human diseases.

Keywords: neutrophil extracellular traps, netosis, receptors, microbial evasion of NETs, autoimmune diseases

1. Introduction

The human organism is constantly exposed to many microbes, most of them being pathogenic microorganisms that can cause life-threatening infections. The host tissues are a good target for colonization and growth of pathogens; however, the immune system developed during the course of evolution, specialized and responsible for protecting against pathogens, effectively prevents infections. Among cells of the immune system, polymorphonuclear cells—neutrophils—deserve a special attention. These cells form the first line of defense against pathogens and their components effectively combat the intruders [1]. Neutrophils are phagocytic cells capable of active migration from blood vessels to the site of infection. Their high efficiency in pathogen killing is possible due to a number of factors with microbicidal activity [2]. The main task of neutrophils is capturing pathogens, i.e., reducing the area of infection and inflammation by effective elimination of microorganisms. To fulfill this task, neutrophils use a number of mechanisms. The best-known one is the phagocytosis that involves capturing pathogenic cells, their internalization and killing in special compartments of neutrophil cells—phagosomes [3]. This mechanism, despite its high efficacy and minimal side-effects for the host, can be insufficient to combat massive bacterial infections or attack of other large-size pathogenic cells. An alternative to phagocytosis is a mechanism described in 2004 by Brinkmann et al., involving web-like structures released into the extracellular space, called neutrophil extracellular traps (NETs) [4]. Morphological changes of neutrophils associated with NET formation ("netosis") involve a number of complex intracellular events. The initial process is a decondensation of nuclear chromatin, released into the extracellular space and forming a backbone of vast NETs. These DNA fibers are decorated with associated nuclear proteins—histones—and proteins released from neutrophil granules such as elastase, myeloperoxidase, lactoferrin, and azurocidin [5, 6].

The netosis is classified as a unique type of cell death, different from apoptosis and necrosis. The mechanism of this process is complex and still incompletely understood although the main processes involved have been identified [7, 8]. NETs can be released in response to many different stimuli, including selected chemical compounds, components of pathogen cells, and whole bacteria, fungi, viruses, and parasites [9]. Released structures are able to capture all of these factors and, in consequence, to reduce the pathogen spreading over the host organism. The NET proteinaceous components, often enzymes, are responsible for killing trapped microorganisms, thus restoring the proper functioning of the host body [10]. However, the same components may also destroy surrounding host cells and tissues or trigger some autoimmune diseases [11].

2. Mechanisms of NET formation

The activation of netosis causes dramatic changes in neutrophil morphology involving the decondensation of chromatin, lysis of granules, and cell membrane rupture and leading to neutrophil death called "programmed suicide" which is a third type of neutrophil defensive action, besides phagocytosis and degranulation [4, 6]. However, the newest studies have shown that in some cases neutrophils use exocytosis to release a part of DNA without any rupture of cell membrane, in a process called "vital netosis." However, this term is still under debate because it is not clear, if neutrophils actually remain alive thereafter [12, 13]. Some reports have suggested that in this fast NET-releasing process it is rather the mitochondrial DNA that is excreted, supporting observations of significantly lower efficiency of NET production in comparison with regular netosis [13]. The classical NET-forming pathway is triggered with massive generation of reactive oxygen species (ROS), resulting from the activity of NADPH oxidase. This ROS-dependent netosis pathway lasts for up to 4 hours, starting from neutrophil activation, and leading to the release of whole nuclear DNA mixed with granular proteins. In contrast, the fast netosis pathway does not require ROS production, leading to a rapid release of NETs within minutes after activation [12].

2.1. Factors that trigger NET production

Netosis can be activated by many compounds, mostly those exposed on the pathogen cell surface. This initial step of NET formation determines the form of released NETs and pathways involved, as well as the intensity and time span of neutrophil response.

The largest group of NET activators are pathogenic Gram-positive and Gram-negative bacteria, but also some fungi (*Aspergillus* spp., *Candida* spp.), as well as viruses (HIV-1, Hantaan virus) and parasites such as *Toxoplasma gondii* and *Leishmania.* Besides microorganisms, numerous chemical factors, including phorbol ester (PMA), hydrogen peroxide, nitric oxide, ionomycin, calcium ions, glucans, mannans, and lipopolysaccharide (LPS), as well as mediators of inflammation such as granulocyte-macrophage colony-stimulating factor (GM-CSF), some interleukins and immune complexes have been identified as potential netosis-triggering factors [9, 11]. Most of them are recognized by neutrophil surface receptors (pattern recognizing receptors, PRRs) that trigger cell signaling for cytokine or chemokine production in order to launch a pathogen-tailored response [14]. Diverse pathogens may be recognized by neutrophils with very similar and overlapping mechanisms.

2.2. Receptors that mediate NET formation

2.2.1. Toll-like receptors

The main PRRs involved in the recognition of pathogens and pathogen-associated molecules are Toll-like receptors (TLRs). Among several TLRs, only TLR2, TLR4, TLR7, and TLR8 have been identified as participating in NET-dependent phenomena. The role of TLR4 in the activation of netosis was confirmed in *Staphylococcus aureus* infection. This receptor plays a great role in the activation of "vital netosis" *in vivo*, cooperating with complement receptor 3 (CR3) [15]. During bacterial sepsis, neutrophils and platelets cooperate in pathogenesis, but the mutual relationship between these cells is still under debate. TLR4, a lipopolysaccharide receptor, seems to mediate the activation of neutrophils by platelets induced by LPS [16].

The other molecule involved in NET triggering via TLRs is high-mobility group box 1 protein (HMGB1). This protein released from dying cells or activated macrophages enhances inflammatory reactions. HMGB1 is a TLR4 agonist, but does not induce the production of ROS by NADPH oxidase, suggesting its involvement in an ROS-independent mechanism of NET formation [17]. On the other hand, an oxidized low density lipoprotein (oxLDL) is able to induce netosis via ROS-dependent pathway, activated by TLR4 and TLR6 receptors [18]. TLR4 was also identified as an important surface recognizing molecule in viruses-activated netosis detected in the lungs of infected hosts. Respiratory syncytial virus (RSV) is responsible for acute bronchiolitis in children under 3 years. This RNA virus exposes a fusion protein (F-protein) on its surface that mediates a fusion of viral envelope with the target cell membrane and also activates NET release using TLR4 mediation [19]. Moreover, F-protein is also recognized by CD14 receptor, which cooperates with TLR4 [20, 21]. A human immunodeficiency virus HIV-1 is captured and killed in NETs formed by neutrophils using TLR7 and TLR8 to recognize viral nucleic acids. Activation of these receptors leads to production of ROS and activation of ROS-dependent netosis pathway [22].

2.2.2. Receptors of complement system

The most commonly identified receptor of complement system that contributes to neutrophil responses is CR3 complex (Mac-1; CD11b/CD18). It has been identified to be involved in NET triggering by different types of pathogenic microorganisms. The role of Mac-1 in NET formation is best known in fungal life-threatening, systemic infections, especially those caused by *Candida albicans*. On the cell wall, *C. albicans* exposes well-characterized compounds, such as β-glucans or mannans, important for activation of netosis [23–25]. The β-glucan particles are bound by Mac-1 allowing to recognize *C. albicans* at early stage of infection, without preliminary opsonization [26]. Some studies have suggested that for *in vitro* activation of netosis by fungal compounds the presence of fibronectin is required [27]. The activation of Mac-1 causes a rapid formation of NETs via the ROS-independent pathway [26, 27]. However, glucans are also able to induce ROS formation through the activation of NADPH oxidase [28].

Mannheimia haemolytica is a bacterium that causes a severe respiratory disease. One of the virulence factors of this pathogen is leukotoxin (LKT), which can lead to the death of many host cells. LKT was also identified as a *M. haemolytica* factor that triggers NET formation via CD18 receptor, but the complete model of this interaction and the regulation of netosis by this toxin are still not fully understood [29].

Aggregatibacter actinomycetemcomitans, as well as *Actinomyces viscosus* and *S. aureus*, also induce NET release by human neutrophils. However, analysis of the complement receptors involved in netosis activated by these bacteria showed that complement receptor 1 (CR1; CD35) rather than CR3 takes part in recognizing the pathogens [30]. However, CR3 seems to be important for the activation of "vital netosis" induced by *S. aureus* [15].

Moreover, some viruses seem to be recognized by neutrophils via complement receptors. Hantaan virus (HTNV), a member of hantaviruses family, causes severe renal and pulmonary pathologies in humans. This virus is known as a potential NET triggering factor that stimulates neutrophils much stronger than Vaccinia virus or LPS. Detailed analysis of mechanisms of neutrophil activation by HTNV indicated that CR3 and CR4 receptors are necessary for activation of netosis using the ROS-dependent pathway [31].

Another microorganism able to induce netosis is a parasite *Eimeria bovis*. Although this pathogen does not cause diseases in humans but causes diseases in animals, e.g., a severe hemorrhagic diarrhea, especially in calves, it is a good example of activation of netosis via CR3 by parasites. The interaction of Mac-1 with *E. bovis* causes a rapid

Ca^{2+}-mobilization and activation of the ROS-dependent netosis pathway with intensive NET expulsion [32].

Complement receptors are also involved in triggering netosis by immune complexes (ICs) that play an important role in many pathogen-associated diseases, as well as noninfectious, autoimmunological diseases. ICs are bound to neutrophil surface by many different receptors, causing activation of the cells. Mac-1 takes part in these interactions leading to NET release. The overall mechanism is still unclear, but it has been confirmed that IC activation of CR3 receptors leads to the increase of NADPH oxidase activity and, thus, to the initiation of ROS-dependent netosis pathway [33].

2.2.3. Fc-receptors

The recognition of opsonized pathogens or antibody-associated foreign molecules is one of key functionalities of the cells of immune system. In the activation of these cells, antibody receptors of the Fc-receptor family are involved. Neutrophil cells express only two types of surface Fc-receptors for IgG molecules, namely, FcγRIIa (CD32a) and FcγRIIIb (CD16b) [34]. Some microorganisms induce NETs only in the presence of autologous serum [15], suggesting a role of Fc-receptors in the activation of netosis, but it has not yet been resolved which receptors, CD32 or CD16, have greater impact. The best-known NET inducers via Fc-receptors are ICs. Some studies showed that FcγRIIa mediates activation of netosis by endocytosis of ICs [35]. However, other authors suggested that FcγRIIa rather promoted phagocytosis and only FcγRIIIb was involved in the induction of netosis [33]. The activation of netosis by CD16 takes about 3 hours with efficient production of ROS, suggesting a similarity to induction of netosis by PMA.

Fc-receptors also seem to participate in NET formation during bacterial infections. The results presented for neutrophils in contact with opsonized *S. aureus* suggest that activation of Fc-receptors modulates netosis [30]. Moreover, coating of bacteria by IgA also enhances NET formation via FcαIR [36].

2.2.4. C-lectin receptors

C-type lectin receptors (CLRs), such as dectin-1, are responsible for recognition of surface exposed β-glucans of pathogens [37, 38]. The role of glucans in activation of netosis as well as the role of dectin-1 receptor in activation of NET formation are still under debate [26]. The involvement of dectin-1 in this process was confirmed for several fungal pathogens, such as *Paracoccidioides brasiliensis* [39]. However, the role of this receptor in the activation of netosis during *C. albicans* infection is still unclear. Some studies seem to support this hypothesis [40], but, on the other hand, Gazendam et al. suggested that unopsonized *C. albicans* cells do not induce netosis via dectin-1 receptor [26]. The role of dectin-1 was also proposed by Li et al. who showed that upon ligand binding a dectin-1 receptor activates Mac-1, and this receptor induces downstream NET formation [41]. Additional evidence presented that dectin-1 may indirectly mediate netosis depending on microbial size. Neutrophils in contact with *C. albicans* hyphae or *Mycobacterium bovis* aggregates were able to release NETs. It was proposed that phagocytosis of microbes mediated by dectin-1 plays the function of microbial size sensor and prevents netosis by downregulation of elastase translocation from granules to the nucleus [42]. The number of *Candida* cells and the level of infection were also proposed to be factors responsible for NET formation [43].

Interestingly, the regulation of NET excretion by PMA, used in *in vitro* models of netosis, occurs without activation of any receptors, but directly by the action on protein kinase C (PKC) [44], an important signal mediator of ROS-dependent netosis pathway [45].

2.3. Netosis pathways

Because many of receptors exposed on neutrophil surface are involved and cause cross-activation in NET triggering processes [46–49], the complete pathway of netosis is still under debate. However, some key steps as well as mediating compounds were proposed to be involved in NET formation and are summarized below; however, the specific processes may vary depending on the trigger type.

The first important mediators of netosis, identified in fungal infections associated with NET release, seem to be Src family kinases and spleen tyrosine kinase (Syk) [31, 40]. Src cooperates with plasma membrane-associated receptors, such as CD11b, CD16, or dectin-1, and causes an activation of Syk. Further, Syk devolves the activation signal downstream to next mediators—phosphoinositide 3-kinase (PI3K)/protein kinase B (Akt), p38 MAPK (mitogen-activated protein kinase), and extracellular signal-regulated kinases (ERK1/2) pathways [33, 50, 51]. Syk is also involved in the activation of protein kinase C (PKC) by PMA [33, 52, 53], without participation of Src, confirming observed bypassing of the receptors by PMA.

Many of the natural NET inducers, activating the receptors mentioned above, lead to the release of calcium ions from endoplasmic reticulum storage into the cytoplasm, increasing PKC activity [54]. PKC is responsible for phosphorylation of $gp91^{phox}$ that can form the functional complex of NADPH oxidase with subsequent ROS generation [55, 56]. ROS are crucial for classical suicidal netosis (ROS-dependent pathway).

Netosis is a different type of neutrophil death in comparison to apoptosis. Although both mechanisms are mutually exclusive, they could be activated by the same receptors. Indeed, neutrophils are able to block apoptosis, to allow for the formation of NETs. A key molecular switch between apoptosis and netosis seems to be protein kinase B. Activation of Akt allows to induce netosis, but inhibition of this enzyme leads to apoptotic cell death. A key role in apoptosis is played by caspases, whose activities are inhibited in netosis [57]. Moreover, ROS may alternatively inactivate caspases favoring autophagy [58].

The role of PI3K in NET formation is still unclear. Some research showed that phosphorylation of PI3K is not important and has no effect on NET formation via activation of CD16 [59]. On the other hand, an activation of netosis by ICs seems to require active PI3K [33]. Moreover, PI3K

http://dx.doi.org/10.5772/intechopen.68443

interplays with Akt [60], as well as influences a nuclear factor kappa-light-chain-enhancer of activated B cells (NF-κB) regulation by production of phosphatidylinositol (3,4,5)-trisphosphate [61]. NF-κB has been identified as a regulatory molecule in netosis [62]. PI3K also regulates the autophagy, an important process in PMA- and oxLDL-induced netosis [18, 58, 63].

The role of ERK1/2 in netosis pathway has also been confirmed [19, 32, 33, 59, 64, 65]. ERK1/2 can be induced by Src/Syk, as well as by TLR receptors via interleukin-1 receptor-associated kinase (IRAK) [66]. These mediators seem to be involved in the ROS-dependent netosis pathway, but the relationship between activation of ERK1/2 and generation of ROS by NADPH oxidase is still unsolved. More probably, ERK1/2 can downstream-activate NADPH oxidase [33, 65] or is itself controlled by ROS [45]. The role of p38 MAPK is also not clear, because some studies showed that inhibition of these kinases has no impact on ROS production and ROS-dependent netosis [33, 67, 68], but other presented an opposite effect [32]. The summary of netosis pathways is schematically presented in **Figure 1**.

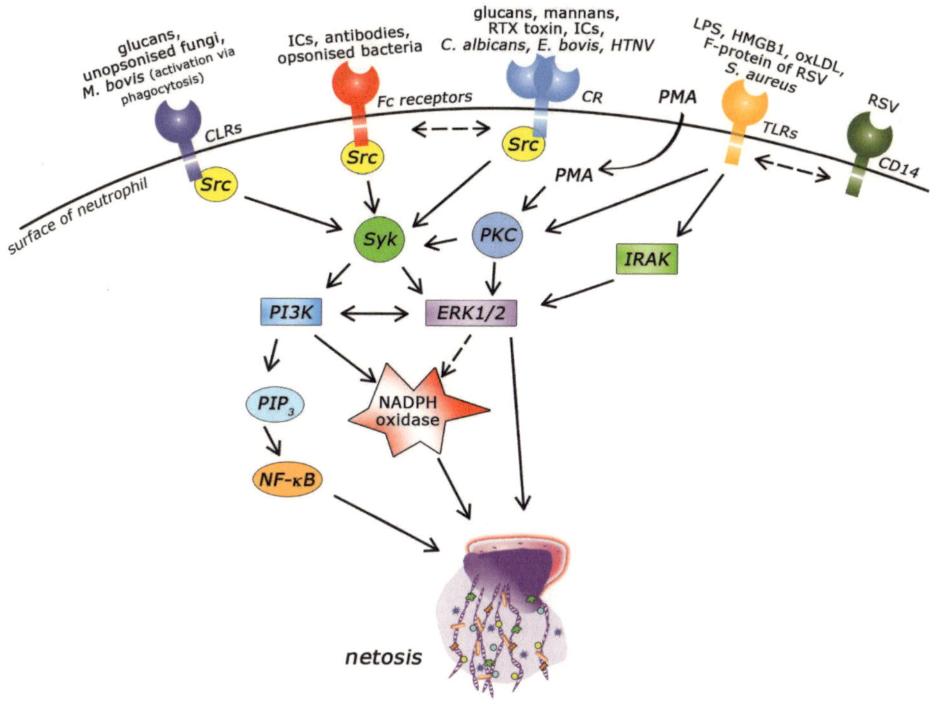

Figure 1. Molecular mechanisms of NET formation. CLRs, C-type lectin receptors; CR, complement receptors; ERK1/2, extracellular signal-regulated kinases; HTNV, Hantaan virus; ICS, immune complexes; IRAK, interleukin-1 receptor-associated kinase; LPS, lipopolysaccharide; PI3K, phosphoinositide 3-kinase; PIP3, phosphatidylinositol (3,4,5)-trisphosphate; PKC, protein kinase C; PMA, phorbol myristate acetate; RSV, respiratory syncytial virus; Src, Src kinase; Syk, spleen tyrosine kinase; TLRs, toll-like receptors.

2.4. Role of ROS in netosis

The first described, classical mechanism of netosis assumed that ROS species play an essential role in netosis (the ROS-dependent pathway) [56]. Indeed, several findings have proven that ROS are key netosis mediators. Patients with chronic granulomatous disease (CGD), caused by a point mutation in gp91^{-phox} subunit of NADPH oxidase, making the enzyme nonfunctional, were more susceptible to infections. Additionally, CGD patients experienced hyper-inflammatory states and sterile inflammations [69, 70]. Moreover, providing ROS from external sources, as well as application to CGD patients a gene therapy, restored the ability of neutrophils to release NETs [8, 46, 71]. Similarly, inhibition of NADPH oxidase by diphenyliodide (DPI) turns off the ability to release NETs [72].

2.5. ROS-independent mechanism of netosis

Little is known about the ROS-independent netosis pathway. NET release without ROS contribution is much faster than the classical netosis. The pathway in which neutrophils remained structurally intact was named as "vital netosis." It can be induced by the same pathogens as those acting in the ROS-dependent manner, e.g., during *Leishmania* parasite infection [12]. Similarly, the induction of NET release in response to glucans of *C. albicans* usually occurs through the ROS-dependent pathway, but in infants, neutrophils release NETs without ROS involvement [73]. Upon contact with *S. aureus* neutrophils release NETs but the web of DNA is released in the exocytosis pathway, without cell membrane rupture. Moreover, NET production was also observed in patients with inactive NADPH oxidase [74]. It was also documented that this type of netosis exploited a release of mitochondrial DNA and an oxidative activity of mitochondrion [13], as well as a small conductance calcium-activated potassium channel 3 (SK3) [75].

2.6. Morphological changes of neutrophils during NET formation

The process of DNA release in the ROS-dependent pathway takes about 1–4 hours and is quite complex. After NADPH oxidase activation, produced ROS probably influence the stability of granules and nuclear envelope. The proteins stored in neutrophil granules—elastase and myeloperoxidase—are moved to the nucleus but the mechanism of their translocation is unknown. In the nucleus, these enzymes contribute to the degradation of linker histones responsible for maintenance of the nuclear structure [55]. They cooperate with next enzyme transferred into the nucleus—peptidyl arginine deiminase 4 (PAD4)—that catalyzes the citrullination of histones, especially H3 and H4. The modification and cleavage of histones lead to the relaxation and decondensation of chromatin, changing the shape and structure of nucleus, and finally causing the disappearance of nuclear membrane [76–78]. DNA is moved into the cytoplasm and mixed with granular proteins such as cathepsin G, proteinase 3, lactoferrin, azurocidin, or with cytoplasmic proteins such as calprotectin [79]. Some research suggests that cytoskeleton also plays an important role in the process of NET formation [46]. At the end of the process, this mixture is released outside the cell. **Figure 2** summarizes all morphological changes during netosis.

http://dx.doi.org/10.5772/intechopen.68443

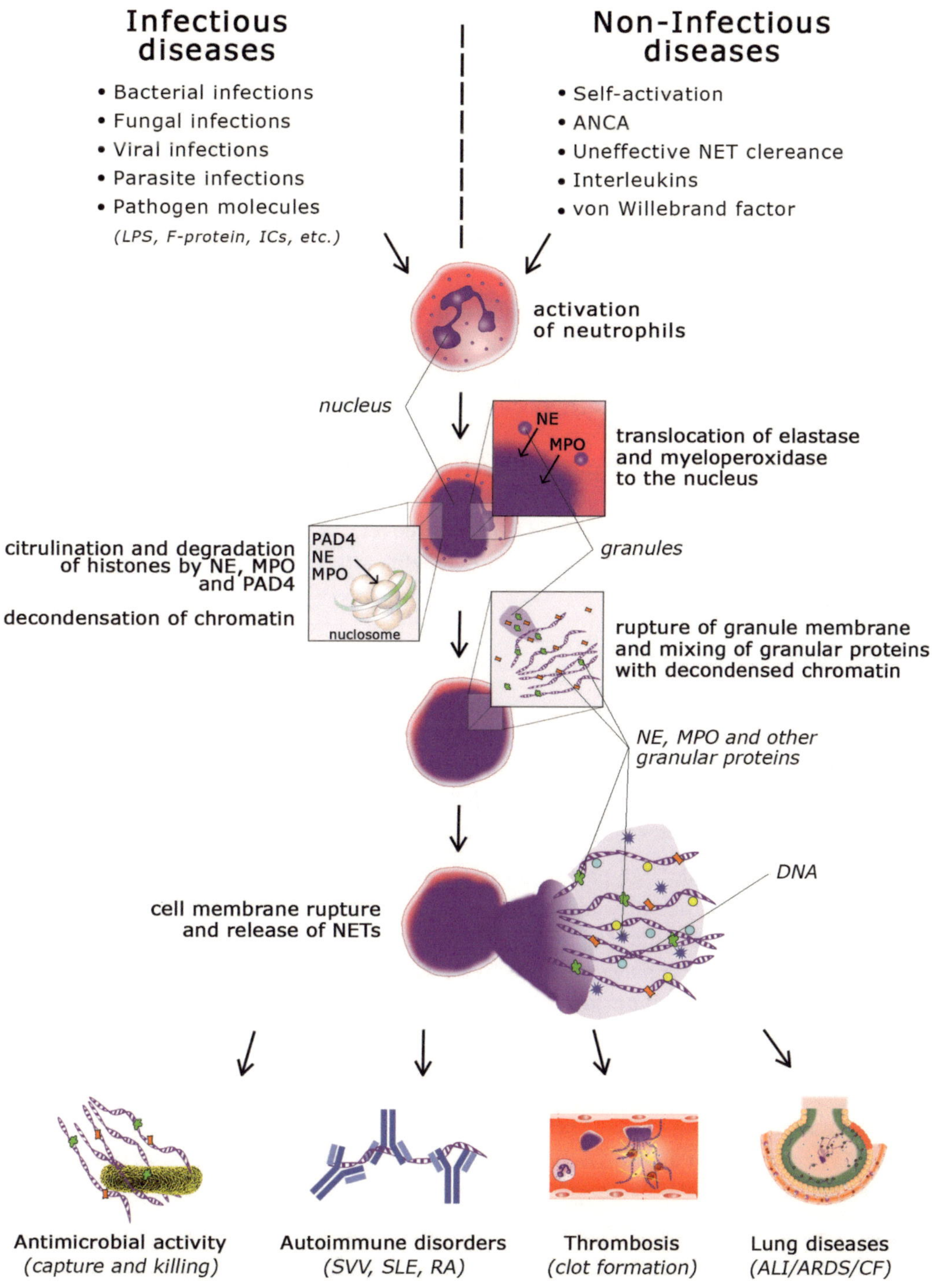

Figure 2. Mechanism of NET formation. ALI, acute lung injury; ARDS, acute respiratory distress syndrome; ANCA, antineutrophil cytoplasmic antibodies; MPO, myeloperoxidase; NE, neutrophil elastase; PAD4, protein arginine deiminase 4; RA, rheumatoid arthritis; SLE, systemic lupus erythematosus; SVV, small vessel vasculitis.

3. Role of NETs in health and diseases

3.1. The microbicidal activity of NETs

The primary role of NETs is the antimicrobial activity, due to the cooperation of several mechanisms and components exposed at the high local concentrations in the NET fibers [55]. The pathogen spreading is limited by entrapment inside NET structure due to electrostatic interactions between the negatively charged DNA backbone and positively charged bacterial compounds localized on their cell surface [6]. Proteinaceous components of NETs are responsible for different types of NET antimicrobial activities. Proteases such as elastase, cathepsin G, and proteinase 3 are able to cleave virulence factors of *Yersinia enterocolitica*, *Shigella flexneri*, *Salmonella Typhimurium*, and other pathogens [4, 80]. The oxidative mechanisms of defense, e.g., the production of aggressive hypochlorous acid by myeloperoxidase, cause massive damages of NET-entrapped pathogens with their membrane and protein oxidation [81, 82]. Histones, as well as antimicrobial peptides such as LL-37 and BPI, also play an important role in pathogen elimination. Peptides derived from histones and LL-37 take part in cell membrane permeabilization or bacterial cell lysis [83–85]. Moreover, NET-associated factors can restrict nutrient supply for microbes, e.g., lactoferrin chelates iron and calprotectin sequesters zinc ions [79, 84].

3.2. Pathogen escape from NETs

Microorganisms that constantly compete with the host defense mechanisms for survival, elaborated also evasion strategies against toxic effects of NETs. The strategies can be divided into three groups, including: (1) an inactivation of NET components responsible for trapping and killing pathogens, (2) a suppression of NET formation and (3) development of resistance mechanisms against antimicrobial components of NETs.

The main NET component, DNA backbone is degraded by bacterial endonucleases, membrane-bound or released into the surrounding milieu. The group of microorganisms that produce such enzymes to avoid the killing activity of NETs includes *S. aureus* whose nuclease influences the bacterial survival and enhances its infectivity in a mouse respiratory tract infection model [86]. The same strategy, leading to decline NET integrity, is also adopted by other bacteria such as *Aeromonas hydrophila* [87], *Escherichia coli* [88], *Leptospira* sp. [89], *Neisseria gonorhoeae* [90], *Streptococcus agalactiae* [91], *Streptococcus pyogenes* [92, 93], *Streptococcus synguinis* [94], *Streptococcus suis* [95], *Vibrio cholerae* [96], and *Yersinia enterocolitica* [88]. *Streptococcus pneumoniae* uses cell-associated endonuclease (EndA) to escape from local entrapment and promote bacterial spreading from lower airways to bloodstream during pneumonia [97]. Also, parasites such as *Leishmania infantum* use nuclease activity to resist the NET activity [98].

Moreover, the production of ROS involved in the initiation and progression of the main netosis pathway can be regulated by bacterial catalase activity in a self-protection process [99].

Other interesting NET evasion strategies were proposed for meningococci [100], which apply the release of outer membrane vesicles for protection of bacteria from binding to NETs and express a high-affinity zinc uptake receptor (ZnuD) to overcome possible ion sequestration by calprotectin, the NET component also known to be involved in *C. albicans* killing during netosis [101]. Moreover, a modification of meningococcal LPS with phosphoethanolamine protects bacteria from bactericidal activity of cathepsin G embedded into NET structures.

The bactericidal activity of another NET component, cathelicidin LL-37, can be abolished by its binding to the surface-expressed M1 protein in *S. pyogenes* [102] or to surface exposed D-alanylated lipoteichoic acid in *S. pyogenes* and *S. pneumoniae*, promoting bacteria survival within NETs [103, 104].

Moreover, *C. albicans* aspartic proteases, secreted during NET formation in response to fungal infection, are able to degrade and inactivate LL-37 [105].

Many bacterial toxins are involved in induction of NETs but some of them are used by bacteria to regulate, in particular to inhibit NET formation [106]. *Bordetella pertussis* causing coughing syndrome adopts adenylate cyclase toxin (ACT) to suppress NET shaping [107]. ACT, after translocation into the host phagocyte, may influence the conversion of ATP to cyclic AMP, that in consequence prolongs neutrophil life span by inhibiting the oxidative burst, being one of the initial signals in NET production. This part of NET formation mechanism is also blocked by streptolysin O (SLO) produced by *S. pyogenes* [108].

In the defense against NET formation, microorganisms can also exploit host signaling as in the case of interleukine-8 (IL-8) production by epithelial cells in response to infection. This chemokine is responsible for neutrophil recruiting and amplification of NET release but *S. pyogenes* can produce a peptidase (SpyCEP) which inactivates IL-8 and reduces NET formation [109].

A more complex strategy, used by *Pseudomonas aeruginosa* [110] or *S. agalactiae* [111], employs molecular mimicry with the acquisition of sialic acid motifs presented on the host cell surface which attenuate NET formation. A comparable, indirect mechanism suppressing NET release has been adopted by *Mycobacterium tuberculosis*. This microorganism that triggers NET release during the first stage of infection activates the production of anti-inflammatory cytokine IL-10 that inhibits TLR-induced ROS production and suppresses further NET generation [112].

Also, viruses can apply this strategy of NET suppression, as demonstrated for HIV-1 envelope glycoprotein [22]. Moreover, Dengue virus serotype-2 can negatively affect NET formation by inhibiting glucose uptake in the ROS-independent mechanism of netosis [113].

On the other hand, conidia *of Aspergillus fumigatus* expose hydrophobin (RodA) that suppresses the formation of NETs [114]. This process is also supported by the production of a positively charged exopolysaccharide—galactosaminogalactan that protects the microorganism from binding by NET components [115]. The polysaccharide capsule negatively modulating NET production that contributes to fungal disease severity was also observed in *Cryptococcus neoformans* infections [116].

Another way to subsist the antimicrobial activity of NETs is applied by *P. aeruginosa* in patients with chronic fibrosis where bacteria during its long-term adaptation can form the resistant biofilm that protects the pathogen [117]. Moreover, *S. pneumoniae* and *Haemophilus influenzae* are even able to embed NETs into biofilm for self-protection [118, 119]. Also, the extracellular matrix components of *C. albicans* biofilm alter its recognition by neutrophils and inhibit release of NETs [43].

All the above mechanisms developed by microorganisms to avoid killing by NETs confirm their ongoing adaptation to the sophisticated processes of host defense.

3.3. Role of nets in noninfectious diseases

Netosis is a process being under control of many mechanisms of activation, but NET fibers seem not to be a target or location specific, and in some cases, their release get out of the control. So, the process can be a double-edged sword, acting also against the host cells. Therefore, NETs seem to play a significant role in several autoimmune disease and disorders, described in detail in others reviews [54, 120].

3.3.1. Lung diseases

A chronic inflammatory state of the lungs leads to the development of acute lung injury (ALI) or acute respiratory distress syndrome (ARDS) [121–123]. The increased permeability of alveoli due to a mechanical ventilation or infection causes an activation of signaling involved in the release of proinflammatory factors by epithelial cells, and in consequence the massive migration and activation of neutrophils.

NET release can be also the trigger of sterile inflammatory state in the lung. Moreover, a lack of surfactant proteins makes a NET clearance difficult. The proteolytic enzymes contained in NETs damage epithelial cells, in consequence releasing more proinflammatory factors. This generates a self-perpetuating mechanism of netosis activation [11, 124, 125].

A similar mechanism was observed in patients with cystic fibrosis (CF), a disease consisting in an increase in mucus viscosity, therefore hindering the clearance of mucus from the airways [126]. The presence of DNA in CF patient sputum increases a mucus viscosity, which correlates with the development of inflammation state and higher migration of neutrophils. The high viscosity of mucus makes it difficult to remove, generating good conditions for bacterial invasion [126, 127].

3.3.2. Autoimmune disorders

Autoimmune diseases including small vessel vasculitis (SVV), systemic lupus erythematosus (SLE), or rheumatoid arthritis (RA) seem to be also associated with uncontrolled release and ineffective clearance of NETs [128–130]. The high amount of NETs and free-circulating DNA causes a production of antineutrophil cytoplasmic antibodies (ANCAs) against DNA and NET-associated proteins such as MPO, cathepsin G, elastase, etc. Autoantibodies to citrullinated proteins (ACPA) seem to be a key pathologic factor in RA. The circulating complexes of antibodies-DNA or antibodies-NET proteins induce multiorgan inflammatory states, as well as inflammations of vessels [11, 13, 131, 132].

3.3.3. Thromvbosis

Deep vein thrombosis (DVT) is a next pathological state mediated by NETs. Neutrophils can be activated in veins by many different factors, including activated platelets, interleukins, proinflammatory cytokines, as well as von Willebrand factor (vWF), released by NET-damaged endothelial cells. NETs, released inside veins, promote the formation of thrombi by binding

http://dx.doi.org/10.5772/intechopen.68443

of necessary blood cells and supporting of clot formation. The uncontrolled netosis can lead to massive DVT and consequently to multiple ischemia [11, 13, 133].

4. Conclusions

The progress in investigation of the fundamental processes leading to activation of netosis during pathogenic infection allows us to better understand the main causes of microbial infections and to consider the consequences of neutrophil responses to the host. All of them pointed out on the possible targets for novel therapeutic approaches regulating immunity responses during microbial infection and counteracting the detrimental NET formation and inflammatory diseases.

Acknowledgements

This work was supported in part by the National Science Center of Poland (grant UMO-2012/05/B/NZ1/00003 awarded to M.R.-K.) and Jagiellonian University (grant K/DSC/003704 awarded to M.Z.).

Author details

Marcin Zawrotniak[1], Andrzej Kozik[2] and Maria Rapala-Kozik[1]*

*Address all correspondence to: maria.rapala-kozik@uj.edu.pl

1 Department of Comparative Biochemistry and Bioanalytics, Faculty of Biochemistry, Biophysics and Biotechnology, Jagiellonian University, Krakow, Poland

2 Department of Analytical Biochemistry, Faculty of Biochemistry, Biophysics and Biotechnology, Jagiellonian University, Krakow, Poland

References

[1] Borregaard N. Neutrophils from marrow to microbes. Immunity. 2010;**33**(5):657–670

[2] Kobayashi SD, DeLeo FR. Role of neutrophils in innate immunity: A systems biology-level approach. Wiley Interdisciplinary Reviews. Systems Biology and Medicine. 2009;**1**(3):309–333

[3] Underhill DM, Ozinsky A. Phagocytosis of microbes: Complexity in action. Annual Review of Immunology. 2002;**20**:825–852

[4] Brinkmann V, Reichard U, Goosmann C, Fauler B, Uhlemann Y, Weiss DS, et al. Neutrophil extracellular traps kill bacteria. Science. 2004;**303**(5663):1532–1535

[5] Matoszka N, Działo J, Tokarz-Deptuła B, Deptuła W. NET and NETosis—New phenomenon in immunology. Postepy Higieny i Medycyny Doswiadczalnej (Online). 2012;**66**:437–445

[6] Brinkmann V, Zychlinsky A. Beneficial suicide: Why neutrophils die to make NETs. Nature Reviews. Microbiology. 2007;**5**(8):577–582

[7] Remijsen Q, Kuijpers TW, Wirawan E, Lippens S, Vandenabeele P, Vanden Berghe T. Dying for a cause: NETosis, mechanisms behind an antimicrobial cell death modality. Cell Death and Differentiation. 2011;**18**(4):581–588

[8] Fuchs Ta, Abed U, Goosmann C, Hurwitz R, Schulze I, Wahn V, et al. Novel cell death program leads to neutrophil extracellular traps. Journal of Cell Biology; 2007 15;**176**(2): 231–241

[9] Guimarães-Costa AB, Nascimento MTC, Wardini AB, Pinto-Da-Silva LH, Saraiva EM. ETosis: A microbicidal mechanism beyond cell death. Journal of Parasitology Research. 2012;**2012**:929743.

[10] Brinkmann V, Zychlinsky A. Neutrophil extracellular traps: Is immunity the second function of chromatin? Journal of Cell Biology. 2012;**198**(5):773–783

[11] Zawrotniak M, Rapala-Kozik M. Neutrophil extracellular traps (NETs)—Formation and implications. Acta Biochimica Polonica. 2013;**60**:277–284

[12] Rochael NC, Guimarães-Costa AB, Nascimento MTC, DeSouza-Vieira TS, Oliveira MP, Garcia e Souza LF, et al. Classical ROS-dependent and early/rapid ROS-independent release of neutrophil extracellular traps triggered by *Leishmania* parasites. Scientific Reports. 2015;**5**:18302

[13] Yang H, Biermann MH, Brauner JM, Liu Y, Zhao Y, Herrmann M. New insights into neutrophil extracellular traps: Mechanisms of formation and role in inflammation. Frontiers in Immunology. 2016;**7**:1–8

[14] Thomas CJ, Schroder K. Pattern recognition receptor function in neutrophils. Trends in Immunology. 2013;**34**(7):317–328

[15] Yipp BG, Petri B, Salina D, Jenne CN, Scott BN V, Zbytnuik LD, et al. Infection-induced NETosis is a dynamic process involving neutrophil multitasking in vivo. Nature Medicine. 2012;**18**(9):1386–1393

[16] Clark SR, Ma AC, Tavener Sa, McDonald B, Goodarzi Z, Kelly MM, et al. Platelet TLR4 activates neutrophil extracellular traps to ensnare bacteria in septic blood. Nature Medicine. 2007;**13**(4):463–469

[17] Tadie J-M, Bae H-B, Jiang S, Park DW, Bell CP, Yang H, et al. HMGB1 promotes neutrophil extracellular trap formation through interactions with Toll-like receptor 4. American Journal of Physiology. Lung Cellular and Molecular Physiology. 2013;**304**(5):L342–L349

[18] Awasthi D, Nagarkoti S, Kumar A, Dubey M, Singh AK, Pathak P, et al. Oxidized LDL induced extracellular trap formation in human neutrophils via TLR-PKC-IRAK-MAPK and NADPH-oxidase activation. Free Radical Biology and Medicine. 2016;**93**:190–203

[19] Funchal GA, Jaeger N, Czepielewski RS, Machado MS, Muraro SP, Stein RT, et al. Respiratory syncytial virus fusion protein promotes TLR-4-dependent neutrophil extracellular trap formation by human neutrophils. PLoS One. 2015;**10**(4):1–14

[20] Kurt-Jones EA, Popova L, Kwinn L, Haynes LM, Jones LP, Tripp RA, et al. Pattern recognition receptors TLR4 and CD14 mediate response to respiratory syncytial virus. Nature Immunology. 2000;**1**(5):398–401

[21] Zanoni I, Ostuni R, Marek LR, Barresi S, Barbalat R, Barton GM, et al. CD14 controls the LPS-induced endocytosis of toll-like receptor 4. Cell. 2011;**147**(4):868–880

[22] Saitoh T, Komano J, Saitoh Y, Misawa T, Takahama M, Kozaki T, et al. Neutrophil extracellular traps mediate a host defense response to human immunodeficiency virus-1. Cell Host and Microbe. 2012;**12**(1):109–116

[23] Boxx GM, Kozel TR, Nishiya CT, Zhang MX. Influence of mannan and glucan on complement activation and C3 binding by *Candida albicans*. Infection and Immunity. 2010;**78**(3):1250–1259

[24] van Bruggen R, Drewniak A, Jansen M, van Houdt M, Roos D, Chapel H, et al. Complement receptor 3, not Dectin-1, is the major receptor on human neutrophils for beta-glucan-bearing particles. Molecular Immunology. 2009;**47**(2–3):575–581

[25] Brogden G, Krimmling T, Adamek M, Naim HY, Steinhagen D, von Köckritz-Blickwede M. The effect of β-glucan on formation and functionality of neutrophil extracellular traps in carp (*Cyprinus carpio* L.). Development and Comparative Immunology. 2014;**44**(2):280–285

[26] Gazendam RP, Van Hamme JL, Tool ATJ, van Houdt M, Verkuijlen PJJH, Herbst M, et al. Two independent killing mechanisms of *Candida albicans* by human neutrophils: Evidence from innate immunity defects. Blood. 2014;**124**(4):590–597

[27] Byrd AS, O'Brien XM, Johnson CM, Lavigne LM, Reichner JS. An extracellular matrix-based mechanism of rapid neutrophil extracellular trap formation in response to *Candida albicans*. Journal of Immunology. 2013;**190**(8):4136–4148

[28] Bonfim-Mendonça PDS, Ratti BA, Godoy JDSR, Negri M, Lima NCA De, Fiorini A, et al. β-Glucan induces reactive oxygen species production in human neutrophils to improve the killing of *Candida albicans* and *Candida glabrata* isolates from vulvovaginal candidiasis. PLoS One. 2014;**9**(9):e107805

[29] Aulik NA, Hellenbrand KM, Klos H, Czuprynski CJ. *Mannheimia haemolytica* and Its leukotoxin cause neutrophil extracellular trap formation by bovine neutrophils. Infection and Immunity. 2010;**78**(11):4454–4466

[30] Palmer LJ, Damgaard C, Holmstrup P, Nielsen CH. Influence of complement on neutrophil extracellular trap release induced by bacteria. Journal of Periodontal Research. 2016;**51**(1):70–76

[31] Raftery MJ, Lalwani P, Krautkrämer E, Peters T, Scharffetter-Kochanek K, Krüger R, et al. β2 integrin mediates hantavirus-induced release of neutrophil extracellular traps. Journal of Experimental Medicine. 2014;**211**(7):1485–1497

[32] Muñoz-Caro T, Mena Huertas SJ aqueline, Conejeros I, Alarcón P, Hidalgo MAMA, Burgos RA, et al. *Eimeria bovis*-triggered neutrophil extracellular trap formation is CD11b-, ERK 1/2-, p38 MAP kinase- and SOCE-dependent. Veterinary Research. 2015;**46**:23

[33] Behnen M, Leschczyk C, Moller S, Batel T, Klinger M, Solbach W, et al. Immobilized immune complexes induce neutrophil extracellular trap release by human neutrophil granulocytes via Fcgamma-RIIIB and Mac-1. Journal of Immunology. 2014;**193**(4):1954–1965

[34] Unkeless JC, Shen Z, Lin CW, DeBeus E. Function of human Fc gamma RIIA and Fc gamma RIIIB. Seminars in Immunology. 1995;**7**(1):37–44

[35] Chen K, Nishi H, Travers R, Tsuboi N, Martinod K, Wagner DD, et al. Endocytosis of soluble immune complexes leads to their clearance by FcygammaRIIIB but induces neutrophil extracellular traps via FcygammaRIIA in vivo. Blood. 2012;**120**(22):4421–4431

[36] Aleyd E, van Hout MWM, Ganzevles SH, Hoeben KA, Everts V, Bakema JE, et al. IgA enhances NETosis and release of neutrophil extracellular traps by polymorphonuclear cells via Fcα receptor I. Journal of Immunology. 2014;**192**(5):2374–2383

[37] Taylor PR, Tsoni SV, Willment JA, Dennehy KM, Rosas M, Findon H, et al. Dectin-1 is required for beta-glucan recognition and control of fungal infection. Nature Immunology. 2007;**8**(1):31–38

[38] Mayadas TN, Cullere X, Lowell CA. The multifaceted functions of neutrophils. Annual Review of Pathology. 2014;**9**:181–218

[39] Bachiega TF ernanda, Dias-Melicio LA, Fernandes RK, de Almeida Balderramas H, Rodrigues DR, Ximenes VF, et al. Participation of dectin-1 receptor on NETs release against *Paracoccidioides brasiliensis*: Role on extracellular killing. Immunobiology. 2016;**221**(2):228–235

[40] Nanì S, Fumagalli L, Sinha U, Kamen L, Scapini P, Berton G. Src family kinases and Syk are required for neutrophil extracellular trap formation in response to β-glucan particles. Journal of Innate Immunity. 2015;**7**(1):59–73

[41] Li X, Utomo A, Cullere X, Choi MM, Milner DA, Venkatesh D, et al. The β-glucan receptor dectin-1 activates the integrin Mac-1 in neutrophils via vav protein signaling to promote *Candida albicans* clearance. Cell Host and Microbe. 2011;**10**(6):603–615

[42] Branzk N, Lubojemska A, Hardison SE, Wang Q, Gutierrez MG, Brown GD, et al. Neutrophils sense microbe size and selectively release neutrophil extracellular traps in response to large pathogens. Nature Immunology. 2014;**15**:1–11

[43] Johnson CJ, Cabezas-Olcoz J, Kernien JF, Wang SX, Beebe DJ, Huttenlocher A, et al. The extracellular matrix of *Candida albicans* biofilms impairs formation of neutrophil extracellular traps. PLOS Pathog. 2016;**12**(9):e1005884

[44] Newton AC. Protein kinase C: Structure, function, and regulation. Journal of Biological Chemistry. 1995;**270**(48):28495–28498

[45] Keshari RS, Verma A, Barthwal MK, Dikshit M. Reactive oxygen species-induced activation of ERK and p38 MAPK mediates PMA-induced NETs release from human neutrophils. Journal of Cellular Biochemistry. 2012;**114**(3):1–24

[46] Neeli I, Dwivedi N, Khan S, Radic M. Regulation of extracellular chromatin release from neutrophils. Journal of Innate Immunity. 2009;**1**(3):194–201

[47] Zhou MJ, Brown EJ. CR3 (Mac-1, alpha M beta 2, CD11b/CD18) and Fc gamma RIII cooperate in generation of a neutrophil respiratory burst: Requirement for Fc gamma RIII and tyrosine phosphorylation. Journal of Cell Biology. 1994;**125**(6):1407–1416

[48] Geijtenbeek TBH, Gringhuis SI. Signalling through C-type lectin receptors: Shaping immune responses. Nature Reviews. Immunology. 2009;**9**(7):465–479

[49] Figueiredo RT, Carneiro LAM, Bozza MT. Fungal surface and innate immune recognition of filamentous fungi. Frontiers in Microbiology. 2011;**2**:1–14

[50] Lowell CA. Src-family and Syk kinases in activating and inhibitory pathways in innate immune cells: Signaling cross talk. Cold Spring Harb Perspect Biology. 2011;**3**(3):1–16

[51] Whitlock BB, Gardai S, Fadok V, Bratton D, Henson PM. Differential roles for alpha(M) beta(2) integrin clustering or activation in the control of apoptosis via regulation of akt and ERK survival mechanisms. Journal of Cell Biology. 2000;**151**(6):1305–1320

[52] Popa-Nita O, Proulx S, Paré G, Rollet-Labelle E, Naccache PH. Crystal-induced neutrophil activation: XI. Implication and novel roles of classical protein kinase C. Journal of Immunology. 2009;**183**(3):2104–2114

[53] Jancinova V, Perecko T, Nosal R, Svitekova K, Drabikova K. The natural stilbenoid piceatannol decreases activity and accelerates apoptosis of human neutrophils: involvement of protein kinase C. Oxidative Medicine Cellular Longevity. 2013;**2013**:136539

[54] Kaplan MJ, Radic M. Neutrophil extracellular traps: double-edged swords of innate immunity. Journal of Immunology. 2012;**189**(6):2689–2695

[55] Papayannopoulos V, Metzler KD, Hakkim A, Zychlinsky A. Neutrophil elastase and myeloperoxidase regulate the formation of neutrophil extracellular traps. Journal of Cell Biology. 2010;**191**(3):677–691

[56] Parker H, Dragunow M, Hampton MB, Kettle AJ, Winterbourn CC. Requirements for NADPH oxidase and myeloperoxidase in neutrophil extracellular trap formation differ depending on the stimulus. Journal of Leukocyte Biology. 2012;**92**(4):841–849

[57] Douda DN, Yip L, Khan MA, Grasemann H, Palaniyar N. Akt is essential to induce NADPH-dependent NETosis and to switch the neutrophil death to apoptosis. Blood. 2014;**123**(4):597–600

[58] Remijsen Q, Vanden Berghe T, Wirawan E, Asselbergh B, Parthoens E, De Rycke R, et al. Neutrophil extracellular trap cell death requires both autophagy and superoxide generation. Cell Research. 2011;**21**(2):290–304

[59] Aleman OR, Mora N, Cortes-Vieyra R, Uribe-Querol E, Rosales C. Differential use of human neutrophil Fc receptors for inducing neutrophil extracellular trap formation. Journal of Immunology Research. 2016;**2016**:2908034

[60] Sekulić A, Hudson CC, Homme JL, Yin P, Otterness DM, Karnitz LM, et al. A direct linkage between the phosphoinositide 3-kinase-AKT signaling pathway and the mammalian target of rapamycin in mitogen-stimulated and transformed cells. Cancer Research. 2000;**60**(13):3504–3513

[61] Ward C, Walker A, Dransfield I, Haslett C, Rossi AG. Regulation of granulocyte apoptosis by NF-kappaB. Biochemical Society Transactions. 2004;**32**(Pt3):465–467

[62] Lapponi MJ, Carestia A, Landoni VI, Rivadeneyra L, Etulain J, Negrotto S, et al. Regulation of neutrophil extracellular trap formation by anti-inflammatory drugs. Journal of Pharmacology and Experimental Therapeutics. 2013;**345**(3):430–437

[63] Kambas K, Mitroulis I, Apostolidou E, Girod A, Chrysanthopoulou A, Pneumatikos I, et al. Autophagy mediates the delivery of thrombogenic tissue factor to neutrophil extracellular traps in human sepsis. PLoS One. 2012;**7**(9):e45427

[64] DeSouza-Vieira T, Guimarães-Costa A, Rochael NC, Lira MN, Nascimento MT, Lima-Gomez P de S, et al. Neutrophil extracellular traps release induced by *Leishmania:* role of PI3Kγ, ERK, PI3Kσ, PKC, and [Ca2+]. Journal of Leukocyte Biology. 2016;**100**:1–9

[65] Hakkim A, Fuchs T a, Martinez NE, Hess S, Prinz H, Zychlinsky A, et al. Activation of the Raf-MEK-ERK pathway is required for neutrophil extracellular trap formation. Nature Chemical Biology. 2011;**7**(2):75–77

[66] Futosi K, Fodor S, Mócsai A. Neutrophil cell surface receptors and their intracellular signal transduction pathways. International Immunopharmacology. 2013;**17**(3):638–650

[67] Detmers PA, Zhou D, Polizzi E, Thieringer R, Hanlon WA, Vaidya S, et al. Role of stress-activated mitogen-activated protein kinase (p38) in beta 2-integrin-dependent neutrophil adhesion and the adhesion-dependent oxidative burst. Journal of Immunology. 1998;**161**(4):1921–1929

[68] Partrick DA, Moore EE, Offner PJ, Meldrum DR, Tamura DY, Johnson JL, et al. Maximal human neutrophil priming for superoxide production and elastase release requires p38 mitogen-activated protein kinase activation. Archives of Surgery. 2000 Feb;**135**(2):219–225

[69] Roxo-Junior P, Simão HML. Chronic granulomatous disease: Why an inflammatory disease? Brazilian Journal of Medical Biological Research = Revista Brasileira Pesquisas medicas e Biologiqas. 2014;**47**(11):924–928

[70] Nishinaka Y, Arai T, Adachi S, Takaori-Kondo A, Yamashita K. Singlet oxygen is essential for neutrophil extracellular trap formation. Biochemical and Biophysical Research Communications. 2011;**413**(1):75–79

[71] Bianchi M, Hakkim A, Brinkmann V, Siler U, Seger R a, Zychlinsky A, et al. Restoration of NET formation by gene therapy in CGD controls aspergillosis. Blood. 2009;**114** (13):2619–2622

[72] Zawrotniak M, Kozik A, Rapala-Kozik M. Selected mucolytic, anti-inflammatory and cardiovascular drugs change the ability of neutrophils to form extracellular traps (NETs). Acta Biochimica Polonica. 2015;**62**(3):465–473

[73] Byrd AS, O'Brien XM, Laforce-Nesbitt SS, Parisi VE, Hirakawa MP, Bliss JM, et al. NETosis in neonates: Evidence of a reactive oxygen species-independent pathway in response to fungal challenge. Journal of Infectious Disease. 2016;**213**(4):634–639

[74] Pilsczek FH, Salina D, Poon KKH, Fahey C, Yipp BG, Sibley CD, et al. A novel mechanism of rapid nuclear neutrophil extracellular trap formation in response to *Staphylococcus aureus*. Journal of Immunology. 2010;**185**(12):7413–7425

[75] Douda DN, Khan M a., Grasemann H, Palaniyar N. SK3 channel and mitochondrial ROS mediate NADPH oxidase-independent NETosis induced by calcium influx. Proceedings of the National Academy of Sciences. 2015;**112**(9):2817–2822

[76] Leshner M, Wang S, Lewis C, Zheng H, Chen XA, Santy L, et al. PAD4 mediated histone hypercitrullination induces heterochromatin decondensation and chromatin unfolding to form neutrophil extracellular trap-like structures. Frontiers in Immunology. 2012;**3**:307

[77] Rohrbach AS, Slade DJ, Thompson PR, Mowen K a. Activation of PAD4 in NET formation. Frontiers in Immunology. 2012;**3**:360

[78] Wang Y, Li M, Stadler S, Correll S, Li P, Wang D, et al. Histone hypercitrullination mediates chromatin decondensation and neutrophil extracellular trap formation. Journal of Cell Biology. 2009;**184**(2):205–213

[79] Urban CF, Ermert D, Schmid M, Abu-Abed U, Goosmann C, Nacken W, et al. Neutrophil extracellular traps contain calprotectin, a cytosolic protein complex involved in host defense against *Candida albicans*. PLoS Pathogens. 2009;**5**(10):e1000639

[80] Averhoff P, Kolbe M, Zychlinsky A, Weinrauch Y. Single residue determines the specificity of neutrophil elastase for *Shigella* virulence factors. Journal of Molecular Biology. 2008;**377**(4):1053–1066

[81] Parker H, Winterbourn CC. Reactive oxidants and myeloperoxidase and their involvement in neutrophil extracellular traps. Frontiers in Immunology. 2012;**3**:424

[82] Klebanoff SJ. Myeloperoxidase: Friend and foe. Journal of Leukocyte Biology. 2005;**77** (5):598–625

[83] Tsao HS, Spinella SA, Lee AT, Elmore DE. Design of novel histone-derived antimicrobial peptides. Peptides. 2009;**30**(12):2168–2173

[84] Papayannopoulos V, Zychlinsky A. NETs: a new strategy for using old weapons. Trends in Immunology. 2009;**30**(11):513–521

[85] Hirsch J. Bactericidal action of histone. Journal of Experimental Medicine. 1958;**108**: 925–944

[86] Berends ETM, Horswill AR, Haste NM, Monestier M, Nizet V, Von Köckritz-Blickwede M. Nuclease expression by *Staphylococcus aureus* facilitates escape from neutrophil extracellular traps. Journal of Innate Immunity. 2010;**2**(6):576–586

[87] Brogden G, von Köckritz-Blickwede M, Adamek M, Reuner F, Jung-Schroers V, Naim HY, et al. β-Glucan protects neutrophil extracellular traps against degradation by *Aeromonas hydrophila* in carp (*Cyprinus carpio*). Fish and Shellfish Immunology. 2012;**33**(4):1060–1054

[88] Möllerherm H, Neumann A, Schilcher K, Blodkamp S, Zeitouni NE, Dersch P, et al. *Yersinia enterocolitica*-mediated degradation of neutrophil extracellular traps (NETs). FEMS Microbiology Letters. 2015;**362**(23):fnv192

[89] Scharrig E, Carestia A, Ferrer MF, Cédola M, Pretre G, Drut R, et al. Neutrophil extracellular traps are involved in the innate immune response to infection with leptospira. PLoS Neglected Tropical Diseases. 2015;**9**(7):e0003927

[90] Juneau RA, Stevens JS, Apicella MA, Criss AK. A thermonuclease of *Neisseria gonorrhoeae* enhances bacterial escape from killing by neutrophil extracellular traps. Journal of Infectious Disease. 2015;**212**(2):316–324

[91] Derré-Bobillot A, Cortes-Perez NG, Yamamoto Y, Kharrat P, Couvé E, Da Cunha V, et al. Nuclease A (Gbs0661), an extracellular nuclease of *Streptococcus agalactiae*, attacks the neutrophil extracellular traps and is needed for full virulence. Molecular Microbiology. 2013;**89**(3):518–531

[92] Buchanan JT, Simpson AJ, Aziz RK, Liu GY, Kristian SA, Kotb M, et al. DNase expression allows the pathogen group A *Streptococcus* to escape killing in neutrophil extracellular traps. Current Biology. 2006;**16**(4):396–400

[93] Chang A, Khemlani A, Kang H, Proft T. Functional analysis of *Streptococcus pyogenes* nuclease A (SpnA), a novel group A streptococcal virulence factor. Molecular Microbiology. 2011;**79**(6):1629–1642

[94] Morita C, Sumioka R, Nakata M, Okahashi N, Wada S, Yamashiro T, et al. Cell wall-anchored nuclease of *Streptococcus sanguinis* contributes to escape from neutrophil extracellular trap-mediated bacteriocidal activity. PLoS One. 2014;**9**(8):e103125

[95] de Buhr N, Neumann A, Jerjomiceva N, von Köckritz-Blickwede M, Baums CG. *Streptococcus suis* DNase SsnA contributes to degradation of neutrophil extracellular traps (NETs) and evasion of NET-mediated antimicrobial activity. Microbiology. 2014;**160**(Pt 2):385–395

[96] Seper A, Hosseinzadeh A, Gorkiewicz G, Lichtenegger S, Roier S, Leitner DR, et al. *Vibrio cholerae* evades neutrophil extracellular traps by the activity of two extracellular nucleases. PLoS Pathogens. 2013;**9**(9):e1003614

[97] Beiter K, Wartha F, Albiger B, Normark S, Zychlinsky A, Henriques-Normark B. An endonuclease allows *Streptococcus pneumoniae* to escape from neutrophil extracellular traps. Current Biology. 2006;**16**(4):401–407

[98] Guimarães-Costa AB, Nascimento MTC, Froment GS, Soares RPP, Morgado FN, Conceição-Silva F, et al. *Leishmania amazonensis* promastigotes induce and are killed by neutrophil extracellular traps. Proceedings of the National Academic Sciences U S A. 2009;**106**(16):6748–6753

[99] Juneau RA, Pang B, Armbruster CE, Murrah KA, Perez AC, Swords WE. Peroxiredoxin-glutaredoxin and catalase promote resistance of nontypeable *Haemophilus influenzae* 86-028NP to oxidants and survival within neutrophil extracellular traps. Infection and Immunity. 2015;**83**(1):239–246

[100] Lappann M, Danhof S, Guenther F, Olivares-Florez S, Mordhorst IL, Vogel U. In vitro resistance mechanisms of *Neisseria meningitidis* against neutrophil extracellular traps. Molecular Microbiology. 2013;**89**(3):433–449

[101] Urban CF, Reichard U, Brinkmann V, Zychlinsky A. Neutrophil extracellular traps capture and kill *Candida albicans* yeast and hyphal forms. Cell Microbiology. 2006;**8**(4):668–676

[102] Lauth X, von Köckritz-Blickwede M, McNamara CW, Myskowski S, Zinkernagel AS, Beall B, et al. M1 protein allows Group A streptococcal survival in phagocyte extracellular traps through cathelicidin inhibition. Journal of Innate Immunity. 2009;**1**(3):202–214

[103] Cole JN, Pence MA, von Köckritz-Blickwede M, Hollands A, Gallo RL, Walker MJ, et al. M protein and hyaluronic acid capsule are essential for in vivo selection of covRS mutations characteristic of invasive serotype M1T1 group A *Streptococcus*. MBio. 2010;**1**(4) e00191-10

[104] Wartha F, Beiter K, Albiger B, Fernebro J, Zychlinsky A, Normark S, et al. Capsule and D-alanylated lipoteichoic acids protect *Streptococcus pneumoniae* against neutrophil extracellular traps. Cell Microbiology. 2007;**9**(5):1162–1171

[105] Rapala-Kozik M, Bochenska O, Zawrotniak M, Wolak N, Trebacz G, Gogol M, et al. Inactivation of the antifungal and immunomodulatory properties of human cathelicidin LL-37 by aspartic proteases produced by the pathogenic yeast *Candida albicans*. Infection and Immunity. 2015;**83**:2518–2530

[106] von Köckritz-Blickwede M, Blodkamp S, Nizet V. Interaction of bacterial exotoxins with neutrophil extracellular traps: impact for the infected host. Frontiers in Microbiology. 2016;**7**:402

[107] Eby JC, Gray MC, Hewlett EL. Cyclic AMP-mediated suppression of neutrophil extracellular trap formation and apoptosis by the *Bordetella pertussis* adenylate cyclase toxin. Infection and Immunity. 2014;**82**(12):5256–5269

[108] Uchiyama S, Döhrmann S, Timmer AM, Dixit N, Ghochani M, Bhandari T, et al. Streptolysin O rapidly impairs neutrophil oxidative burst and antibacterial responses to group A Streptococcus. Frontiers in Immunology. 2015;**6**:581

[109] Zinkernagel AS, Timmer AM, Pence MA, Locke JB, Buchanan JT, Turner CE, et al. The IL-8 protease SpyCEP/ScpC of group A Streptococcus promotes resistance to neutrophil killing. Cell Host and Microbe. 2008;**4**(2):170–178

[110] Khatua B, Bhattacharya K, Mandal C. Sialoglycoproteins adsorbed by *Pseudomonas aeruginosa* facilitate their survival by impeding neutrophil extracellular trap through siglec-9. Journal of Leukocyte Biology. 2012;**91**(4):641–655

[111] Carlin AF, Uchiyama S, Chang Y-C, Lewis AL, Nizet V, Varki A. Molecular mimicry of host sialylated glycans allows a bacterial pathogen to engage neutrophil Siglec-9 and dampen the innate immune response. Blood. 2009;**113**(14):3333–3336

[112] Hahn S, Giaglis S, Chowdhury CS, Chowdury CS, Hösli I, Hasler P. Modulation of neutrophil NETosis: interplay between infectious agents and underlying host physiology. Seminars in Immunopathology. 2013;**35**(4):439–453

[113] Moreno-Altamirano MMB, Rodríguez-Espinosa O, Rojas-Espinosa O, Pliego-Rivero B, Sánchez-García FJ, Rodríguez-Espinosa O, et al. Dengue virus serotype-2 interferes with the formation of neutrophil extracellular traps. Intervirology. 2015;**58**(4):250–259

[114] Bruns S, Kniemeyer O, Hasenberg M, Aimanianda V, Nietzsche S, Thywissen A, et al. Production of extracellular traps against *Aspergillus fumigatus* in vitro and in infected lung tissue is dependent on invading neutrophils and influenced by hydrophobin RodA. PLoS Pathogens. 2010;**6**(4):e1000873

[115] Lee MJ, Liu H, Barker BM, Snarr BD, Gravelat FN, Al Abdallah Q, et al. The fungal exopolysaccharide galactosaminogalactan mediates virulence by enhancing resistance to neutrophil extracellular traps. PLoS Pathogens. 2015;**11**(10):e1005187

[116] Rocha JDB, Nascimento MTC, Decote-Ricardo D, Côrte-Real S, Morrot A, Heise N, et al. Capsular polysaccharides from *Cryptococcus neoformans* modulate production of neutrophil extracellular traps (NETs) by human neutrophils. Scientific Reports. 2015 Jan 26;**5**:8008

[117] Young RL, Malcolm KC, Kret JE, Caceres SM, Poch KR, Nichols DP, et al. Neutrophil extracellular trap (NET)-mediated killing of *Pseudomonas aeruginosa*: evidence of acquired resistance within the CF airway, independent of CFTR. PLoS One. 2011 ;**6**(9):e23637

[118] Hong W, Juneau RA, Pang B, Swords WE. Survival of bacterial biofilms within neutrophil extracellular traps promotes nontypeable *Haemophilus influenzae* persistence in the chinchilla model for otitis media. Journal of Innate Immunity. 2009;**1**(3):215–224

[119] Reid SD, Hong W, Dew KE, Winn DR, Pang B, Watt J, et al. *Streptococcus pneumoniae* forms surface-attached communities in the middle ear of experimentally infected chinchillas. Journal of Infectious Disease. 2009;**199**(6):786–794

[120] Mitsios A, Arampatzioglou A, Arelaki S, Mitroulis I, Ritis K. NETopathies? Unraveling the dark side of old diseases through neutrophils. Frontiers in Immunology. 2017;**7**:1–13

[121] Cheng OZ, Palaniyar N. NET balancing: a problem in inflammatory lung diseases. Frontiers in Immunology. 2013;**4**:1

[122] Grommes J, Soehnlein O. Contribution of neutrophils to acute lung injury. Molecular Medicine. 2011;**17**(3–4):293–307

[123] Narasaraju T, Yang E, Samy RP, Ng HH, Poh WP, Liew A-A, et al. Excessive neutrophils and neutrophil extracellular traps contribute to acute lung injury of *Influenza pneumonitis*. The American Journal of Pathology. 2011;**179**(1):199–210

[124] Douda DN, Jackson R, Grasemann H, Palaniyar N. Innate immune collectin surfactant protein D simultaneously binds both neutrophil extracellular traps and carbohydrate ligands and promotes bacterial trapping. Journal of Immunology. 2011;**187**(4):1856–1865

[125] Nayak A, Dodagatta-Marri E, Tsolaki AG, Kishore U. An insight into the diverse roles of surfactant proteins, SP-A and SP-D in innate and adaptive immunity. Frontiers in Immunology. 2012;**3**:131

[126] Henke MO, Ratjen F. Mucolytics in cystic fibrosis. Paediatric Respiratory Reviews. 2007;**8**(1):24–29

[127] Kaynar a M, Shapiro SD. NET loss of air in cystic fibrosis. Nature Medicine. 2010;**16**(9):967–969

[128] Sangaletti S, Tripodo C, Chiodoni C, Guarnotta C, Cappetti B, Casalini P, et al. Neutrophil extracellular traps mediate transfer of cytoplasmic neutrophil antigens to myeloid dendritic cells toward ANCA induction and associated autoimmunity. Blood. 2012;**120**(15):3007–3018

[129] Kessenbrock K, Krumbholz M, Schönermarck U, Back W, Gross WL, Werb Z, et al. Netting neutrophils in autoimmune small-vessel vasculitis. Nature Medicine. 2009;15(6):623–625

[130] Crispín JC, Liossis SC, Kis-Toth K, Lieberman LA, Kyttaris VC, Juang Y, et al. Pathogenesis of human systemic lupus erythematosus: recent advances. Trends in Molecular Medicine. 2010;16(2):47–57

[131] Kallenberg CGM, Heeringa P, Stegeman CA. Mechanisms of disease: Pathogenesis and treatment of ANCA-associated vasculitides. Nature Clinical Practice. Rheumatology. 2006;**2**(12):661–670

[132] Diamantopoulos AP. Extracellular neutrophil traps: A novel therapeutic target in ANCA-associated vasculitis? Frontiers in Immunology. 2013;**4**:24

[133] Fuchs TA, Brill A, Wagner DD. Neutrophil extracellular trap (NET) impact on deep vein thrombosis. Arteriosclerosis, Thrombosis, and Vascular Biology. 2012;**32**(8):1777–1783

Chapter 2

Beneficial and Deleterious Effects of Neutrophil Extracellular Traps on Infection

Maximina B. Moreno-Altamirano,

Christian E. Cruz-Gómez and Lluvia E. López-Luis

Additional information is available at the end of the chapter

http://dx.doi.org/10.5772/intechopen.68634

Abstract

Polymorphonuclear neutrophils (PMNs) are the most abundant leukocytes in the blood and are considered as the first line of innate immune defence against infectious diseases. However, PMN cells have a crucial function in both innate and adaptive immune responses. Neutrophils have several mechanisms to control pathogens, and one of them is their capability to form neutrophil extracellular traps (NETs) that may control infection. NETs have the capacity to trap microorganisms, kill them, or avoid their dissemination. The aim of this chapter is to provide a comprehensive review on NETs, the cells that produce them, and some of the mechanisms involved in their formation, their role in the immune response, and the pros and cons of NETs, focusing mainly on infectious diseases.

Keywords: neutrophil extracellular traps (NETs), neutrophils, bacteria, viruses, infectious diseases

1. Introduction

The polymorphonuclear neutrophils (PMNs), first reported by Ilya Ilych Mechnikov, better known as Élie Metchnikoff, are the most abundant leukocytes (60%) in the blood. These PMNs are considered as the first line of innate immune response against infectious agents [1]. Later on, Carl Friedrich Claus suggested the term of phagocytosis for the function of these cells. Studies aimed at the fully understanding of their properties and functions in controlling a variety of pathogens are still in progress. Research on neutrophils has focused on their phagocytic capacity and, more recently, on their role as neutrophil extracellular traps (NETs) forming cells, in innate and adaptive immunity.

When neutrophils fail to kill invading pathogens by the classical phagocytosis mechanism, PMNs can accomplish this function by neutrophil extracellular traps (NETs), a process reported as a novel form of cell death called NETosis, which is dependent of the generation of reactive oxygen species [2–5]. Neutrophils forming NETs have been demonstrated by activating neutrophils with phorbol myristate acetate (PMA), interleukin 8 (IL-8), lipopolysaccharide (LPS), or under contact of neutrophils with Gram-negative and Gram-positive bacteria.

NETosis induction has also been described for viral infections, and some of the signaling pathways involved have been analyzed, finding the involvement of pathogen-associated molecular patterns (PAMPs), TLR-4, TLR-7, and TLR-8. Rodríguez-Espinosa et al. have shown that NETs formation takes place in two separate metabolic steps: the first one involves chromatin decondensation, which is independent of external glucose and glycolysis, whereas the second, which involves the chromatin release, is a process that is dependent on external glucose and glycolysis [6].

2. Understanding the process of NETs formation

The neutrophil extracellular traps (NETs) structures were described as another type of neutrophil cell death, different from apoptosis and necrosis. The research field on NETs has steadily been growing since 2004, when Brinkmann et al. reported for the first time this new function of activated neutrophils, demonstrating, by electron microscopy, that, when neutrophils are in the presence of bacteria, fungi, protozoa, or viruses, they acquire the capacity to form fibrillary structures, resembling nets or webs. These structures are composed mainly of nuclear material, chromatin fibers with diameters of 15–17 nm containing DNA decorated with neutrophil elastase (NE), myeloperoxidase (MPO), cathepsin G, proteinase 3 (PR3), high-mobility group protein B1 (HMGB-1), tryptase or antimicrobial peptide LL37, histones, and cytoplasmic proteins such as histones H1, H2A, H2B, H3, H4, G, lactoferrin, and gelatinase, among others [7].

Two mechanisms for the formation of NETs have been described: the suicide or lytic and vital NETosis [8]. In the first case, NETs release results from the activation of PMN by IL-8 or chemical compounds, such as phorbol myristate acetate (PMA). PMA activates neutrophils through the protein kinase C (PKC) and follows the Raf-MEK-ERK mitogen-activated protein kinase signaling pathway; the enzyme nicotinamide adenine dinucleotide phosphate (NADPH) oxidase induces the translocation of elastase from the cytosolic granules to the inner nucleus, helping the rupture of the chromatin through histones. Induction of NETs with PMA by this mechanism can be observed from 30 min post-activation and, by 6–8 h post-activation, a high number of extracellular traps (ETs) are well formed (**Figure 1**).

In contrast, vital NETosis has been demonstrated following pathogen recognition by host pattern recognition receptors (PRRs). Gram-negative bacteria products, such as lipopolysaccharide

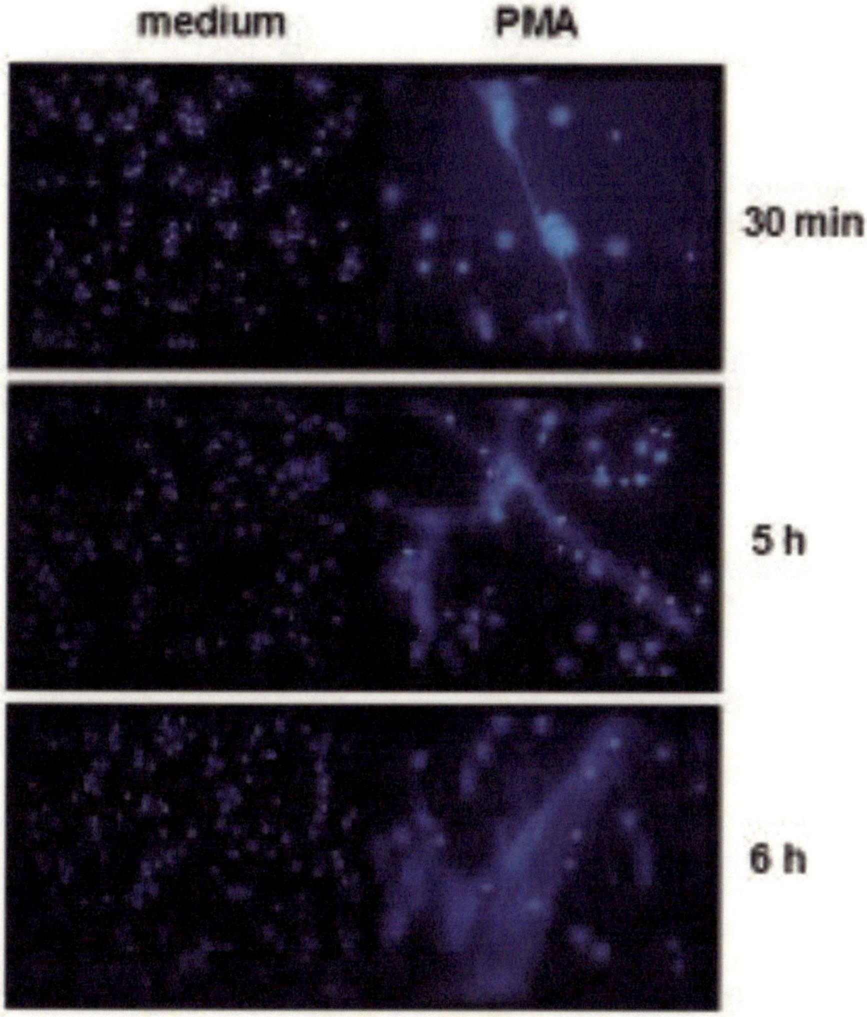

Figure 1. Human peripheral blood neutrophils non-activated and activated with PMA (100 ng/ml) for different lengths of time. Neutrophil extracellular traps formation starts by 30 min post-activation; extracellular traps are more extended by 6 h post-activation (photographs taken by Moreno-Altamirano).

(LPS), activate neutrophils, by the ligation of TLRs (TLR-4 in the case of LPS), inducing the liberation of NETs. In the case of Gram-positive bacteria, the complement receptor 3 (CR3) and TLR-2 are required to induce vital NETosis; platelets are also inducers of vital NETosis, through CD11a. This mechanism maintains the external membrane integrity and thus the function of neutrophils, until cells are devoid of nucleus [7, 8].

A third mechanism for the induction of NETs, recently reported, is through autophagy [9, 10]. It is worth mentioning that neutrophils are not the only cells that form extracellular traps (ETs), and other immune cells, such as mast cells, eosinophils, and macrophages, can also release ETs. Although the molecular principles underlying the formation of ETs by mast cells [11], eosinophils [12], and monocytes/macrophages [13] are similar to those observed in neutrophils, there are some notable disparities. The most remarkable mechanism of ET formation has been described in eosinophils. In these cells, ETs are formed by both nuclear and mitochondrial DNAs, in a reactive oxygen species (ROS)-dependent manner.

Neutrophil extracellular traps are able to capture microorganisms trap microorganisms, killing them or not, this much depends on the type of pathogen involved. NETs are produced by the neutrophils of mice, humans, and some other animals, and can be induced by chemical compounds, bacteria, fungi, protozoa, and viruses. The role of NETs in viral infections is not yet clear. However, some viruses induce the release of NETs [14, 15].

While some viruses are immobilized and inactivated by NETs, others such as HIV induce the production of an IL-10-like protein that inhibits the formation of NETs [15], and dengue virus inhibits PMA-induced formation of NETs. Interestingly, neutrophils seem to be arrested at the chromatin decondensation step, failing to liberate NETs, thus suggesting a metabolic-related mechanism of NETs inhibition [16].

Controversy surrounding neutrophil extracellular traps as a host defense mechanism makes it necessary to analyze how NETs limit the growth of various infectious agents, whereas, apparently, they have no effect on others. On the other hand, how NETs may cause damage and autoimmune diseases also needs to be investigated.

3. Neutrophil extracellular traps in bacterial infections

Several mechanisms have been proposed to explain how NETs control bacterial infection. NETs bind to both Gram-negative and Gram-positive bacteria, precluding bacterial mobilization and dissemination, and some bacteria are killed extracellularly by NETs, due to their high content of serine proteases [17]. Some bacteria and their interaction with NETs are summarized as follows:

Bordetella pertussis, the causative agent of pertussis or whooping cough, is a Gram-negative aerobic bacterium that infects the respiratory tract and inhibits the host's immune system by mean of its virulent factors, such as pertussis toxin, filamentous hemagglutinin, pertactin, fimbria, and tracheal cytotoxin. The pertussis toxin inhibits G protein coupling that regulates the adenylate cyclase-mediating conversion of ATP to cAMP. This event induces macrophages and neutrophils to convert the ATP to cAMP by intracellular eukaryotic calmodulin, causing disturbances in cellular signaling mechanisms and thus preventing phagocytosis and an efficient control of the pathogen. The formation of NETs induced by *B. pertussis* is NADPH oxidase dependent [18].

Escherichia coli, the causative bacteria of several pathologies, including bacterial sepsis, is a Gram-negative bacterium. NETs formation helps to control infection by trapping and killing the bacteria and avoiding dissemination to other organs. The proposed mechanisms for the formation of NETs depend on the bacteria strain and its pathogenesis. In the case of *E. coli* involved in liver sepsis, the infection can be controlled by histones H2B or by activating the intravascular NETs release through the integrin lymphocyte function-associated antigen 1 (LFA-1) [19, 20].

Klebsiella pneumoniae, the common cause of pneumonia, is caused by this aerobic Gram-negative bacillus. The role of NETs in the killing of *K. pneumoniae* has been investigated; this bacterium is not sufficient to induce NETs in neutrophils *ex vivo*, but it is in the lungs of a murine model. Adenosine A2B receptor deficiency improves survival and enhances bacterial killing and clearance due to NETs formation [21]. In addition, TREM-1 also mediates NETs formation, leading to a bactericidal effect and the control of infection [22].

Leptospira interrogans is the causative agent of leptospirosis. The pathogen spirochetes Gram-negative belongs to the Leptospiraceae family and to the genus Leptospira. Leptospirosis is an emerging zoonotic disease, affecting animals and humans in the world, but most frequently in tropical and subtropical countries. This disease is associated with exposure of individuals to wild or farm animals. Scharrig et al. [23], demonstrated for the first time the induction of NETs in human *ex vivo* and murine *in vivo* models, when incubating human neutrophils with Leptospira interrogans LI-130 (LIC). This research group observed that the bacteria number, the pathogenicity, and viability were relevant factors for induction of NETs; however, the motility of bacteria was not. Entrapment of LIC in the NETs resulted in Leptospira death. Pathogenic, but not saprophytic, Leptospira exerted nuclease activity, thus degrading the DNA, concluding that formation of NETs was dependent on bacterial concentration, pathogenicity, and viability, but not motility, and that NETs could trap and kill *Leptospira interrogans* [23].

Mannheimia haemolytica, the causative agent of bovine respiratory disease complex (BRD), is a Gram-negative bacterium that induces a severe pleuropneumonia in bovine animals, where neutrophils play a key role in the pathogenesis. Extracellular traps are induced in neutrophils and macrophages exposed to the bacteria or to their virulent factor, leucotoxin (LKT) [24].

Mycobacterium bovis, the etiological agent of bovine tuberculosis, is a Gram-positive bacterium, with a worldwide distribution, easily transmitted to bovine animals and to humans. The extracellular traps formation has been demonstrated in neutrophils and macrophages. Neutrophils can sense the size of pathogens, and based on their size, neutrophils are induced to undergo necrosis, apoptosis, or NETosis [25].

Mycobacterium tuberculosis is the causative agent of tuberculosis. Ramos-Kichik et al. showed that both *M. tuberculosis* and *Mycobacterium canetti* can induce NETs, which trap but not kill these mycobacterial species [26]. On the other hand, the mycobacterium-derived early secretory antigenic target protein of 6 kDa (ESAT-6) can induce the formation of NETs in *M. tuberculosis*-infected neutrophils [27].

Pseudomonas aeruginosa, the causative agent of the cystic fibrosis lung disease, is a Gram-negative opportunistic bacterium. The formation of NETs in the context of *P. aeruginosa* is controversial, and evidence that NETs may have a major anti-*P. aeruginosa* activity must be clarified [28].

Salmonella typhimurium, a Gram-negative bacterium, induces the release of NETs, and some of their components, such as histones (H2), have bactericidal activity, whereas others, such as elastase, can degrade virulence factors, as in the case of the alpha toxin [7, 29].

Shigella flexneri, a Gram-negative bacterium, induces the release of NETs. *S. flexneri* is trapped by NETs and killed via the neutrophil elastase; virulence factors such as IcsA and IpaB are degraded by the neutrophil elastase [7].

Staphylococcus aureus is some Gram-positive bacteria that cause sepsis. The role of NETs in controlling a *S. aureus* infection could be through the antimicrobial proteins associated to these, the bactericidal effect of H2 histones, the antimicrobial action of the cathelicidin LL-37, and neutrophil proteases that decrease the secretion of the alpha-toxin (α-toxin). The virulence factors LukGH and PVL help to induce the release of NETs. The *S. aureus*-induced release of NETs is an NADPH oxidase-independent process [30].

Staphylococcus epidermidis belongs to the group of coagulase-negative straphylococci. It is a quite common colonizer of healthy mice and human skin. It is a part of "normal" skin flora and plays a beneficial role in cutaneous niche. However, in immunocompromised patients, there is a high risk of developing infection mainly due to catheters use in hospitals. The exoprotein of *S. epidermidis*, the delta-toxin, PMSs (Phenol-Soluble Moduline-gamma) cooperates with host antimicrobial peptides to help kill pathogens of the group A of Streptococcus (GAS). In 2010, Cogen et al. [31] reported that the exoprotein phenol-soluble-moduline -gamma (PSMs) (δ-toxin) can induce NETs formation. The authors demonstrated a direct binding of δ-toxin to LL-37, CRAMP, hBD2, hBD3, as well as DNA.

Streptococcus spp. are Gram-positive bacteria that include non-pathogenic commensal strains and highly virulent pathogenic strains. The pathogenic strains express virulent factors that allow them to evade the immune system. *Streptococcus pneumoniae* infection leads to pneumonia and invasive diseases such as meningitis and bacteremia, whereas *Streptococcus pyogenes* is the major causative agent of Severe Group A Streptococcal Infections. *S. pneumoniae* and *S. pyogenes* induce the formation of NETs. However, these bacteria have evolved mechanisms that allow them to modulate the formation of NETs. Neutrophils, on the other hand, have evolved a NETs release mechanism in response to *Streptococcus*-derived virulence factors. The *S. pyogenes* virulent factor M1 decreases the induction of NETs while conferring bacterial resistance to be killed by NETs. The *S. pyogenes*-derived M1 exotoxin induces the formation of NETs, by associating with fibrinogen and forming a complex that stimulates neutrophils. Formation of NETs contributes to the pathogen elimination [32].

In summary, this review shows that in response to bacterial stimuli, neutrophils get activated and form NETs that may trap and kill invading bacteria. Besides the "classical" way of clearing pathogens by phagocytosis and intracellular exposure to bactericidal compounds, this novel mechanism of neutrophil extracellular killing plays an important role in primary host defense. Moreover, knowledge on the mechanisms of bacterial adaptation to evade the immune system could be used in the medical practice. For instance, DNases inhibitors can be used as potential therapeutics, to prevent degradation of NETs by Group A Streptococcus DNases. In the future, therapeutics aimed at the maintenance of NETs could be used to help clear bacterial infections.

http://dx.doi.org/10.5772/intechopen.68634

4. Neutrophil extracellular traps in parasitic infections

Neutrophil extracellular traps have been broadly studied in regard to bacteria. The role of NETs against protozoa, however, has just recently been analyzed. Protozoa can induce NETs in neutrophils and macrophages, and knowledge on the mechanisms at play is just emerging.

In 2011, Abdi Abdallah [33] reported that human neutrophils produce NETs in response to stimulation with *Plasmodium falciparum* trophozoites, *Leishmania braziliensis,* and *Toxoplasma gondii* tachyzoites. *In vitro* experiments have demonstrated the presence of NETs upon bovine neutrophils stimulation with *Eimeria bovis* sporozoites, in human neutrophils after stimulation with promastigotes of *Leishmania donovani, Leishmania major, Leishmania chagasi, or L. amazonensis* amastigotes. A brief description of the mechanism involved in protozoa-induced NETs formation is next described.

Toxoplasma gondii is an obligated intracellular parasite that causes toxoplasmosis in immunocompromised individuals. In immunocompetent individuals, however, the immune system usually keeps the parasite from causing illness. *Toxoplasma gondii* tachyzoites induce the release of NETs by activating the MEK-ERK signaling pathway. NETs can trap *Toxoplasma gondii* tachyzoites, eliminating about 25% of them as parasite trapping avoids their dissemination [34].

Plasmodium falciparum, an intracellular parasite, causes malaria. It is estimated that this parasite infects between 215 and 659 million humans per year, worldwide. Malaria is transmitted to humans by the bite of Anopheles mosquitoes. *P. falciparum* sporozoites develop into merozoites and enter into erythrocytes. Studies conducted in Nigerian children infected with *P. falciparum* showed NETs structures with trapped trophozoites, and in their blood, infected and non-infected erythrocytes were also observed [35–37].

Eimeria bovis. This parasite is the causative agent of enteritis in cattle, and NETs formed are released upon stimulation with *E. bovis* sporozoites. This parasite stage of *E. bovis* seems to be a better inducer of NETs than PMA. NETs have been shown to diminish infection by parasite immobilization and also by parasite killing, although to a lesser extent [38, 39].

Leishmania spp. These protozoal parasites are the causative agents of leishmaniosis, and the leishmaniosis model has been quite useful in studies on the role of NETs at the early stages of the disease. The promastigote has been identified as the main parasite stage as inducer of NETs. Promastigotes and amastigotes numbers diminish upon NETs release. Histones H2A and H2B are the main inducers of NETs, and these are highly toxic for the parasite. The promastigote form of the parasite can evade the NETs by means of its 3′ nucleotidase, enzyme that degrades the DNA, allowing *Leishmania* spp. to escape from being killed by NETs [40].

In 2015, Rochael et al. analyzed the role of reactive oxygen species, neutrophil elastase, myeloperoxidase, and the PAD4 enzyme in the formation of NETs by *L. amazonensis* promastigotes, in human cells. These authors observed that *Leishmania* promastigotes promote a redox disbalance in neutrophils. The exposure of neutrophils to H_2O_2 induces histone deamination mediated by PAD4, and the redox disbalance takes place independently of the parasite viability, thus suggesting that *Leishmani*a induces the production of ROS through an NADPH oxidase-dependent mechanism [41].

Leishmania as well as *Staphylococcus aureus* induces the release of NETs by an early and rapid mechanism, through an ROS-independent pathway, which is inhibited by an elastase inhibitor and, in contrast to classic NETosis, is not affected by chloramidina. PAD4 activity is only relevant during classic NETosis. Promastigotes viability after treatment of parasites with a NETs-rich supernatant, obtained from either the early and rapid or the classic pathways, shows a reduction of about 42% [41].

As previously described, the interaction of *Leishmania amazonensis* with human neutrophils leads to the release of NETs, which trap and kill the parasite. However, the signaling pathways leading to *Leishmania*-induced NETosis are still under study. However, it has been shown that PI3K, independently of protein kinase B, has a role in parasite-induced NETosis. The main PI3K isoforms involved are PI3Kγ and PI3Kδ. Activation of ERK downstream of PI3Kγ is necessary to trigger an ROS-dependent parasite-induced NETosis. Pharmacological inhibition of protein kinase C also significantly decreases parasite-induced NETs release. Intracellular calcium, regulated by PI3Kδ, represents an alternative ROS-independent pathway of NETosis stimulation by *L. amazonensis*. Finally, intracellular calcium mobilization and reactive oxygen species generation are the major regulators of parasite-induced NETosis. These results contribute to a better understanding of the signaling behind *Leishmania*-induced NETosis [42].

Entamoeba histolytica. This protozoan parasite causes amebiasis, amoebic colitis, and hepatic abscess. Since this parasite is too large to be phagocytosed, Avila et al. [43] analyzed the possibility that this parasite induces the formation of NETs. These authors demonstrated that the amoeba lipopeptidophosphoglycan induces NETs in a dose-dependent manner. NETs can be readily observed 15 min after stimulation; however, by 1 h at a 1:20 infection ratio, NETs occupy a whole microscopic field. NETs induction depends on trophozoite integrity; 30 min after contact with NETs, trophozoites show no changes in size or morphology, and this contact does not have any effect on viability or growth at any time of incubation. On the other hand, it was observed that *E. histolytica* is resistant to cathelicidin LL-37. Resistance to NETs exposure was also studied upon addition of a proteases inhibitor, resulting in that proteases are not responsible for trophozoite resistance to NETs. However, the use of ethylene glycol-bis(β-aminoethyl ether)-N,N,N′,N′-tetraacetic acid (EGTA), a divalent anion chelant, had a deleterious effect in the growth of amoebas that were in contact with NETs, suggesting that trophozoites may have DNAse activity, responsible for its resistance to NETs [43].

Ávila et al. demonstrated that parasite growth could only take place in the absence of a calcium chelant, since enzymes such as trophozoite DNAsas require calcium. This provides an example of NETs inhibition by parasite-produced enzymes. *Entamoeba histolytica* is one of the main parasites that cause stomach diseases worldwide. It causes intestine and liver invasion, associated with the recruitment of large amounts of neutrophils at the early stages of infection [43].

http://dx.doi.org/10.5772/intechopen.68634

5. Neutrophil extracellular traps in fungus infection

5.1. *Aspergillus fumigatus* and *Aspergillus nidulans*

The *Aspergullus fumigatus* species is isolated in 80% of invasive aspergillosis patients. Chronic granulomatosis disease patients, whose cells are not able to undergo respiratory burst, are highly susceptible to infection by fungus of the *Aspergillus* genus such as *A. nidulans*. This indicates the important role of the host respiratory burst, which is also involved in the formation of NETs.

Recent reports highlight the importance of glucosaminoglycans (GAG) in *A. fumigatus* virulence. GAG helps the formation of biofilms and purified soluble GAG induces NK cell-mediated apoptosis of neutrophils, *in vitro*.

Fungus resistance to neutrophil-mediated killing positively correlates with the amount of cell wall-associated GAG. Fungus GAG content functions as the analog of bacterial capside, enhancing resistance to NETs. Although the mechanism by which exopolysaccharides mediate resistance to NETs has not been defined, it is suggested that GAG may inhibit hyphae-NETs binding, perhaps due to the repulsion between the *Aspergillus* exopolysaccharide positive charges and the positive charges present in the NETs antimicrobial peptides and histones [44, 45]. *Aspergillus* induces respiratory burst through its glycosaminoglycans that activate the NAPDH oxidase system, yielding ROS and activating classic NETosis activation [44].

5.2. *Candida albicans*

In 2006, Urban et al. showed that NETs can kill *Candida albicans* in any of its two forms, yeast, which is the proliferating form, or the filamentous, which is the invasive and tissue destructive form. This was corroborated by means of electronic microscopy which showed NETs and *C. albicans* hyphae co-localization, which suggested that hyphae are trapped by NETs, thus controlling the infection [46, 47].

Experiments aimed at analyzing the effect that PMA-activated NETs have on *C. albicans* showed that 20–30% of fungus dies after exposure to NETs [46].

The analysis of the components present in the neutrophil granules that may be responsible for the killing of *Candida albicans* showed that histones are not accountable for this. It was determined that human Neutrophil Granular Extract (hNGE) is responsible for the fungus death, in a dose-dependent manner. These granules contain Bactericidal/permeability-increasing (BPI) protein lactoferrin, and defensins. It appears that the release of NETs is related to the microorganism cell wall composition; the binding of microorganisms by NETs is mediated by ionic forces and thus, the fact that the *Candida* wall contains numerous proteins with phosphodiester bonds with negative charges makes it likely that they bind the positive charges of proteins and histones present in NETs [48].

Kenno et al. analyzed the induction of NETs by *Candida albicans*, and they corroborated that the distinctive forms of *Candida albicans*, hyphae or yeast, may induce NETs. These authors found that hyphae induce higher amounts of NETs than the yeast form, after 4 hours of incubation. *Candida albicans* hyphae stimulate cells through autophagy but not ROS, whereas the yeast form induces NETs through autophagy and ROS. *C. albicans β-glycans* induce NETosis by an ROS-independent mechanism [49, 50].

5.3. Cryptococcus neoformans

In 2015, Rocha et al. described that the opportunistic fungus *Cryptococcus neoformans*, which possesses a glucuronoxylomannan (GMX)-containing capside, precludes this fungus to be phagocytosed by neutrophils. These authors also demonstrated that the acapsular strain of *Cryptococcus neoformans*, which harbor glucuronoxylomannogalactan (GMXgal), is capable of inducing NETs. In contrast, the capsular strain does not induce the release of NETs [51].

The release of NETs by the acapsular strain of *Cryptococcus neoformans* is dependent on ROS generation and the PAD4 enzyme. The capsular strain also inhibits PMA-induced NETs formation [51]. NETs release has also been observed in response to *Cryptococcus gattii* stimulation.

Analysis of *Cryptococcus neoformans* susceptibility to acapsular strain-induced NETs showed that NETs diminished colony-forming units (CFUs) by 80% in the capsular strain and by 54% in the case of the acapsular strain. For this, it is necessary that NETs contain MPO.

Paracoccidioides brasiliensis and *Paracoccidioides lutzii* are fungi of the *Paracoccidioides* genus that cause high mortality and morbidity by the systemic mycosis Paracoccidioidomycosis (PCM), mostly in Latin American countries. Della Coletta et al. [52] have investigated the role of neutrophil extracellular traps on these fungi, reporting the formation of NETs by the yeasts *P. brasiliensis* and *P. luttzii*.

6. Neutrophil extracellular traps in viral infections

Viruses have an extraordinary ability to evade the immune system, and the innate immune system is regarded as the first line of defense. Innate immune cells recognize a wide variety of pathogens through their pattern-recognition receptors (PRRs) that include Toll-like receptors (TLRs), NOD-like receptors (NLRs), and RIG-like receptors (RLRs) that recognize pathogen-associated molecular patterns (PAMPs). Several PRRs recognize viral ligands such as TLR-3, TLR-7, TLR-8, RIG-1, and MDA5, and the activation of these PRRs induces the synthesis of antiviral interferons (types I and II), tumor necrosis factor α, interleukin-15, and interleukin-18 [53–55].

The role of NETs in the control of several bacterial infections has been broadly analyzed. However, research on their role in viral infections remains scarce. It has recently been shown that viral infections or virus-derived molecules may act as strong inducers of NETs. Several viruses that induce the formation of NETs have been identified. In some cases, NETs neutralize the viral particles by the MPO or the granule-derived defensins, associated to NETs. The α-defensin protein directly inhibits the influenza virus replication and protein synthesis [56].

Some viruses, such as those of the herpesvirus family, contain proteins with endonuclease activity, so they can degrade NETs and allow viral escape and dissemination. NETs antiviral activity consists in the sequestering of viral particles, thus preventing fusion of viruses with target cells and direct neutralization of virions. It is worth mentioning that viruses do not necessarily infect the neutrophils. However, neutrophils can sense viral particles through their PRRs or via secondary signals produced upon infection of other host cells. The use of secondary signals to induce the release of NETs has important advantages in the context of viral infections [56, 57].

Viruses that induce the release of NETs *in vitro* do so under a non-productive infection of neutrophils. In the case of HIV-1, neutrophils sense this virus by endosomal PRRs that detect viral nucleic acid via TLR-7 and TLR-8, and then undergo NETosis. The respiratory syncytial virus (RSV) induces NETosis through TLR-4. Hantaviruses induce NETs formation by signaling through β_2 integrins. Influenza virus A can stimulate neutrophils directly to release NETs. Viruses also produce NETs indirectly without engagement of the PRRs expressed by neutrophils. Interleukin-8 (IL-8) triggers NETosis. Although NETs formation by viruses is now well established, it is not so clear how NETs contribute to antiviral immunity. In some viruses, as in a mouse model of poxvirus infection, induction of NETs with LPS prior to infection strongly reduced the number of virus-infected liver cells, and this protective effect was reversed by DNAse treatment. Noroviruses can be reduced by their binding to histone H1. Some viral mechanisms counteract NETs formation, as for HIV-1 envelope glycoprotein which stimulates DCs to produce cellular IL-10 through dendritic cell-specific ICAM-grabbing non-integrin (DC-SIGN), IL-10 is an immunosuppressive cytokine that, among other functions, inhibits TLR-induced ROS production (54). IL-10 homologs have been found in the genome of large DNA viruses that include ubiquitous human virus, such as human cytomegalovirus (HCMV) and Epstein-Barr virus (EBV). Kaposi's sarcoma-associated herpesvirus (KSHV) impairs the release of NETs, and dengue virus serotype-2 can arrest NETs release by interfering with glucose uptake [6]. Taken together, these findings suggest that virus-induced release of NETs may help to control viral dissemination by direct and indirect mechanisms, whereas, at the same time, viral evasion mechanisms target the formation of NETs.

In 2015, Moreno-Altamirano et al. [16] demonstrated that dengue virus serotype-2 inhibits PMA-induced formation of NETs, arresting neutrophils at the chromatin de-condensation step which, based on a previous report [6], suggests that DENV-2 inhibits the formation of NETs by interfering with glucose uptake and glycolysis.

7. Conclusion

Anti-microbial properties of NETs have been shown for bacteria, protozoa, fungus, and virus. Understanding how neutrophil extracellular traps (NETs) limit the growth of some infectious agents, whereas, apparently, they have no effect on others, and how NETs may cause tissue damage and contribute to the development of pathologies, such as autoimmune diseases, will help to exploit their anti-pathogen properties at full, and to limit their pathogenic effects, in clinical settings. It is quite likely that this research field will continue providing exciting findings.

Author details

Maximina B. Moreno-Altamirano*, Christian E. Cruz-Gómez and Lluvia E. López-Luis

*Address all correspondence to: bertha.moreno.altamirano@gmail.com

Department of Immunology, National School of Biological Sciences (ENCB), National Politechnic Institute (IPN), Mexico City, Mexico

References

[1] Kaufmann SH. Immunology's foundation: The 100-year anniversary of the Nobel Prize to Paul Ehrlich and Elie Metchnikoff. Nature Immunology. 2008;**9**:705-712

[2] Nathan C. Neutrophils and immunity: Challenges and opportunities. Nature Reviews Immunology. 2006;**6**:173-182

[3] Fuchs TA, Abed U, Goosmann C, et al. Novel cell death program leads to neutrophil extracellular traps. Journal of Cell Biology. 2007;**176**:231-241

[4] Gupta AK, Joshi MB, Philippova M, et al. Activated endothelial cells induce neutrophil extracellular traps and are susceptible to NETosis-mediated cell death. FEBS Letters. 2010;**584**:3193-3197

[5] Neeli I, Khan SN, Radic M. Histone deimination as a response to inflammatory stimuli in neutrophils. Journal of Immunopharmacology. 2008;**180**:1895-1902

[6] Rodríguez-Espinosa O, Rojas-Espinosa O, Moreno-Altamirano MM, López-Villegas EO, Sánchez-García FJ. Metabolic requirements for neutrophil extracellular traps formation. Immunology. 2015;**145**(2):213-224. DOI: 10.1111/imm.12437

[7] Brinkmann V, Reichard U, Goosmann G, Fauler B, Uhlemann Y, Weiss DS, Weinrauch Y, Zychlinsky A. Neutrophil extracellular traps kill bacteria. Science. 2004;**30**:1532-1535

[8] Yipp BG, Kubes P. NETosis: How vital is it? Blood. 2013;**122**(16):2784-2794

[9] Yang H, Biermann MH, Brauner JM, Liu Y, Zhao Y, Hermann M. New insights into neutrophil extracellular traps: Mechanisms of formation and role in inflammation. Frontiers in Immunology. 2016;**7**:302

[10] Remijsen Q, Berghe TW, Wirawan E, Asselbergh B, et al. Neutrophil extracellular traps cell death requires both autophagy and superoxide generation. Cell Research. 2011;**21**:290-304

[11] von Köckritz-Blickwede, Goldmann O, Thulin P, Heinemann K, Norrby-Teglund A, Rohde M, Medina E. Phagocytosis-independent antimicrobial activity of mast cells by means of extracellular trap formation. Blood. 2008;**111**(6):3070-3080

[12] Yousefi S, Gold JA, Andina N, Lee JJ, Kelly AM, Kozlowski E, Schmid I, Straumann A, Reichenbach J, Gleich GJ, Simon HU. Catapult-like release of mitochondrial DNA by eosinophils contributes to antibacterial defense. Nature Medicine. 2008;**14**(9):949-953

[13] Chow OA, von Kôckritz-Blickwede M, Bright AT, Hensler ME, Zinkernagel AS, Cogen AL, Gallo RL, Monestier M, Wang Y, Glass CK, Nizet V. Statins enhance formation of phagocyte extracellular traps. Cell Host & Microbe. 2010;**8**:445-454

[14] Wardini AB, Guimaraes-Costa AB, Nascimento MT, Nadaes NR, Danelli MG, Mazur C, Benjamim CF, Saraiva EM, Pinto-da-Silva LH. Characterization of neutrophil extracellular traps in cats naturally infected with feline leukemia virus. Journal of General Virology. 2010;**91**:259-264

[15] Saitoh T, Komano J, Saitoh Y, Misawa T, Takahama M, Kozaki T, Uehata T, Iwasaki H, Omori H, Yamaoka S, Yamamoto N, Akira S. Neutrophil extracellular traps mediate a host defense response to human immunodeficiency virus-1. Cell Host & Microbe. 2012;**12**:109-116

[16] Moreno-Altamirano MM, Rodríguez-Espinosa O, Rojas-Espinosa O, Pliego-Rivero B & Sánchez-García FJ. Dengue virus Serotype-2 interferes with the formation of neutrophil extracellular traps. Intervirology. 2015;**58**:250-259

[17] Kumar V, Sharma A. Neutrophils: Cinderella of innate immune system. International Immunopharmacology. 2010;**10**:1325-1334

[18] Eby JC, Gray MC, Hewlett EL. Cyclic AMP-mediated suppression of neutrophil extracellular trap formation and apoptosis by the *Bordetella pertussis* adenylate cyclase toxin. Infection and Immunity. 2014;**82**(12):5256-5269

[19] Marin-Esteban V, Turbica I, Dufour G, Semiramoth N, Gleizes A, Gorges R, Beau I, Servin AL, Lievin-Le Moal V, Sandré C, Chollet-Martin S. Afa/Dr diffusely adhering escherichia coli strain C1845 induces neutrophil extracellular traps that kill bacteria and damage human Enterocyte-Like cells. Infection and Immunity. 2012;**80**(5):1891-1899

[20] McDonald B, Urrutia R, Yipp BG, Jenne CN, Kubes P. Intravascular neutrophil extracellular traps capture bacteria from the bloodstream during sepsis. Cell Host & Microbe. 2012;**12**(3):324-33

[21] Papayannopoulos V, Metzler KD, Hakkim A, Zychlinsky A. Neutrophil elastase and myeloperoxidase regulate the formation of neutrophil extracellular traps. The Journal of Cell Biology. 2010;**191**(3):677-691

[22] Barletta KE, Cagnina RE, Burdick MD, Linden J, Mehrad B. Adenosine A2B receptor deficiency promotes host defenses against Gram-Negative bacterial pneumonia. American Journal of Respiratory and Critical Care Medicine. 2012;**186**:1044-1050

[23] Scharrig E, Carestia A, Ferrer MF, Cédola M, Pretre G, Drut R, Picardeau, Mirta Schattner M, Gómez RM. Neutrophil extracellular traps are involved in the innate immune response to infection with leptospira. PLoS Neglected Tropical Diseases. 2015;**9**(7):3927

[24] Aulik NA, Hellenbrand KM, Czuprynski CJ. Mannheimia haemolytica and its leukotoxin cause macrophage extracellular trap formation by bovine macrophages. Infection and Immunity. 2012;**80**(5):1923-1933

[25] Branzk N, Lubojemska A, Hardison SE, Wang Q, Gutierrez MG, Brow GD, Papayannopoulos V. Neutrophils sense microbe size and selectively release neutrophil extracellular traps in response to large pathogens. Nature Immunology. 2014;**15**(11):1017-1025

[26] Ramos-Kichik V, Mondragón-Flores R, Mondragón-Castelán M, Gonzalez-Pozos S, Muñiz-Hernandez S, Rojas-Espinosa O, Chacón-Salinas R. Estrada-Parra S, Estrada-García I. Neutrophil extracellular traps are induced by Mycobacterium tuberculosis. Tuberculosis. 2009;**89**:29-37

[27] Francis RJ, Butler RE, Stewart GR. Mycobacterium tuberculosis ESAT-6 is a leukocidin causing Ca^{2+} influx, necrosis and neutrophil extracellular trap formation. Cell Death and Disease. 2014;**5**:1474

[28] Yuen J, Pluthero FG, Douda DN, Riedl M, Cherry A, Ulanova M, Kahr WH, Palaniyar N, Licht C. NETosing neutrophils activate complement both on their own NETs and bacteria via alternative and Non-alternative pathways. Frontiers in Immunology. 2016;**7**:137

[29] Manda A, Pruchniak MP, Araźna M, Demkow UA. Neutrophil extracellular traps in physiology and pathology. Central European Journal of Immunology. 2014;**39**(1):116-121

[30] Malachowa N, Kobayashi SD, Freedman B, Dorward DW, DeLeo FR. Staphylococcus aureus leukotoxin GH promotes formation of neutrophil extracellular traps. The Journal of Immunology. 2013;**191**:6022-6029

[31] Cogen AL, Yamasaki K, Muto J, Sánchez KM, Crotty Alexander I, Tanios J, et al. Staphylococcus epidermidis antimicrobial delta-toxin (phenol-soluble modulin-gamma) cooperates with host antimicrobial peptides to kill group a streptococcus. PLoS One. 2010;**5**:e8557. DOI: 10.1371/journal.pone.0008557

[32] Köckritz-Blickwede Maren von, Blodkamp S, Nizet V. Interaction of bacterial exotoxins with neutrophil extracellular traps: Impact for the infected host. Frontiers in Microbiology. 2016;**7**:402

[33] Abi Abdallah D, Denkers E. Neutrophils cast extracellular traps in response to protozoan parasites. Frontiers in Immunology. 2012;**3**:382

[34] Abi Abdallah D, Lin C, Ball C, King M, Duhamel G, Denkers E. *Toxoplasma gondii* triggers release of human and mouse neutrophil extracellular traps. Infection and Immunity. 2011;**80**(2):768-777

[35] Baker VS, Imade GE, Molta NB, Tawde P, Pam SD, Obadofin MO, Sagay SA, Egah DZ, Iya D, Afolabi BB, Baker M, Ford K, Ford R, Roux KH, Keller 3rd TC. Cytokine-associated neutrophil extracellular traps and antinuclear antibodies in *Plasmodium falciparum* infected children under six years of age. Malaria Journal. 2008;**7**:41. DOI: 10.1186/1475-2875-7-41

[36] Camicia G. Neutrophil extracellular traps: A 2-faced host defense mechanism. Medicina Clinica. 2012;**140**:2

[37] Gabelloni M, Sabbione F. Trampas extracelulares de neutrófilos: Una novedosa estrategia antiinfecciosa empleando moléculas antimicrobianas largamente conocidas. Química Viva. 2013;**1**:13

[38] Behrendt JH, Ruiz A, Zahner H, Taubert A, Hermosilla C. Neutrophil extracellular trap formation as innate immune reactions against the apicomplexan parasite *Eimeria bovis*. Veterinary Immunology and Immunopathology. 2010;**133**(1)1-8

[39] Muñoz Caro T, Mena Huerta SJ, Conejeros I, Alarcón P, et al. Eimeria bovis-triggered neutrophil extracellular trap formation is CD11b-, ERK1/2-, p38, MAP Kinase- and SOCE-dependent. Veterinary Research. 2015;**46**:23. DOI: 10.1186/s13567-015-0155-6

[40] Guimaraes-Costa A, DeSouza-Vieira T, Paletta-Silva R, Freitas-Mesquita A, Meyer-Fernandes J, Saraiva E. 3′-Nucleotidase/nuclease activity allows leishmania parasites to escape killing by neutrophil extracellular traps. Infection and Immunity. 2014;**82**(4):1732-1740

[41] Rochael N, Anderson B, Guimarães-Costa A, Nascimento MTC, DeSouza-Vieira T, Oliveira M, Garcia e Souza L, Oliveira M, Saraiva E. Classical ROS-dependent and early/rapid ROS-independent release of neutrophil extracellular traps triggered by leishmania parasites. Scientific Reports. 2015;**5**:18302. DOI: 1038/srep18302

[42] DeSouza-Vieira T, Guimarães-Costa A, Rochael NC, Lira MN, Nascimento MT, Lima-Gomez PS, Mariante RM, Persechini PM, Saraiva EM. Neutrophil extracellular traps release induced by *Leishmania*: role of PI3Kγ, ERK, PI3Kσ, PKC, and [Ca^{2+}]. Journal of Leukocyte Biology. 2016;**100**(4):801-810

[43] Ávila E, Salaiza N, Pulido J, Rodríguez M, Díaz-Godínez C, Laclette J, Becker I, Carrero J. Entamoeba histolytica trophozoites and lipopeptidophosphoglycan trigger human neutrophil extracellular traps. PLoS One. 2016;**11**(7):e0158979

[44] Lee M, Liu H, Barker B, Snarr B, Gravelat F, Al Abdallah Q, Gavino C, Baistrocchi S, Ostapska H, Xiao T, Ralph B, Solis N, Lehoux M, Baptista S, Thammahong A, Cerone R, Kaminskyj S, Guiot M, Latgé J, Fontaine T, Vinh D, Filler S, Sheppard D. The fungal exopolysaccharide galactosaminogalactan mediates virulence by enhancing resistance to neutrophil extracellular traps. PLoS Pathogens. 2015;**11**(10):e1005187

[45] Bruns S, Kniemeyer O, Hasenberg M, et al. Production of extracellular traps against Aspergillus fumigatus in vitro and in infected lung tissue is dependent on invading neutrophils and influenced by hydrophobin RodA. PLoS Pathogens. 2010;**6**(4):e1000873. DOI: 10.1371/journal.ppat.1000873

[46] Urban CF, Reichard U, Brinkmann V, Zychlinsky A. Neutrophil extracellular traps capture and kill Candida albicans yeast and hyphal forms. Cellular Microbiology. 2006;**8**(4):668-676

[47] Chad JJ, Cabezas-Olcoz J, Kernien J, et al. The extracellular matrix of *Candida albicans* biofilms impairs formation of neutrophil extracellular traps. PLoS Pathogens. 2016;**12**(9):e 1005884

[48] Urban CF, Ermert D, Schmid M, Abu.Abed U, Goosman C, Nacken W, Brinkmann V, Jungblut PR, Zychlinsky A. Neutrophil extracellular traps contain, a cytosolic protein complex involved in host defense against *Candida albicans*. PLoS Pathogens. 2009;5:e1000639. DOI: 10.1371/journal.ppat.1000639

[49] Kenno S, Perito S, Mosci P, Vecchiarelli A, Monari C. Autophagy and reactive oxygen species are involved in neutrophil extracellular traps release induced by *C. albicans* morphotypes. Frontiers in Microbiology. 2016;**7**:879

[50] Byrd AS, O'Brien XM, Johnson CM. Lavigne LM, Reichner JS. An extracellular matrix-based mechanism of rapid neutrophil extracellular trap formation in response to *Candida albicans*. Journal of Immunology. 2013;**190**:4136-4148

[51] Rocha J, Nascimento M, Decote-Ricardo D, Côrte-Real S, Morrot A, Heise N, Nunes M, Previato J, Mendonça-Previato L, DosReis G, Saraiva E, Freire-de-Lima C. Capsular polysaccharides from *Cryptococcus neoformans* modulate production of neutrophil extracellular traps (NETs) by human neutrophils. Scientific Reports. 2015;**5**:8008

[52] Della Coletta AM, Bachiega TF, Carvalho de Ouaglia e Silva J, Soares AM, De Faveri J, Marques SA, et al. Neutrophil extracellular traps identification in tegumentary lesions of patients with paracoccidioidomycosis and different patterns of NETs generation in vitro. PLoS. 2015;**9**(9):e0004037. DOI: or/10.1371/journal.pntd.0004037

[53] Akira S. Innate immunity and adjuvants. Philosophical Transactions of the Royal Society B: Biological Science. 2011;**366**:2748-2755

[54] McGill J, Heusel JW, Legge KL. Innate immune control and regulation of influenza virus infections. Journal of Leukocyte Biology. 2009;**86**:803-812

[55] Salvatore M, García-Sastre A, Ruchala P, Lehrer RI, Chang T, et al. Alpha-Defensin inhibits influenza virus replication by cell-mediated mechanism(s). Journal of Infectious Diseases. 2007;**196**:835-843

[56] Jenne CN, Wong CHY, Zemp FJ, McDonald B, Rahman MM, et al. Neutrophils recruited to sites of infection protect from virus challenge by releasing neutrophil extracellular traps. Cell Host & Microbes. 2013;**13**:169-180

[57] Koupenova M, Vitseva O, Mackay CR, Beaulieu LM, Benjamin EJ, Mick E, et al. Platelet-TLR7 mediates host survival and platelet count during viral infection in the absence of platelet-dependent thrombosis. Blood. 2014;**124**:791-802

Chapter 3

The Role of Neutrophil Extracellular Traps in Post-Injury Inflammation

Eszter Tuboly, Gabrielle D. Briggs and Zsolt J. Balogh

Additional information is available at the end of the chapter

http://dx.doi.org/10.5772/intechopen.68906

Abstract

Polymorphonuclear (neutrophil) granulocytes (PMNs) are an essential part of the innate immune responses and key instigators and effectors of the underlying pathological mechanisms (endothelial damage, interstitial histolysis, cytokine production, phagocytosis) leading to post-injury inflammation and secondary tissue injury. In 2004, the formation of neutrophil extracellular traps (NETs) was identified as an additional defence mechanism of PMN against microbes. The understanding of complex regulation of neutrophil functions and NET formation is essential for differentiating between healthy and pathological inflammatory response, which frequently determines if patient recovers uneventfully or develops catastrophic complications. Recent discoveries have revealed the potential role of NETs in the pathogenesis of a wide range of non-infectious diseases, including post-injury sterile inflammation. In such conditions, both spontaneous NET formation and impaired NETosis are documented. In this chapter, we review the evidence for the role of NETs in post-injury inflammation, the key molecular and cellular participants in pathological NET formation, the clinical relevance of NETs in post-injury complications and the therapeutic potential of NET inhibition/clearance.

Keywords: neutrophil granulocyte, PMN, post-injury inflammation, neutrophil extracellular traps, trauma, injury, multiple organ failure

1. Introduction

Despite recent improvements in the care of the injured, severe trauma remains a major burden on our society, resulting in the annual death of more than five million people worldwide (World Health Organisation. Injuries and violence: the facts. 2014. http://www.who.

int/violence_injury_prevention/key_facts/en/ Accessed 9 May 2016). Tissue injury, traumatic shock and subsequent resuscitation and surgical interventions lead to localised and systemic inflammatory responses. Polymorphonuclear (neutrophil) granulocytes (PMNs) are an essential part of the innate immune responses and key instigators and effectors of the underlying pathological mechanisms (endothelial damage, interstitial histolysis, cytokine production, phagocytosis) leading to post-injury inflammation and secondary tissue injury. In 2004, the formation of neutrophil extracellular traps (NETs) was identified as an additional defence mechanism of PMN against microbes [1]. Since the initial description of their antibacterial function, a series of studies reported the existence of NETs in response to various types of sterile inflammations including traumatic injury [2–5]. The precise triggers, contributions and outcomes of NETs in trauma patients are not well understood. Given the significant clinical impact of sterile inflammation in these patients, understanding the role of NETosis may identify novel biomarkers or therapeutic strategies to minimise post-injury tissue damage and hyperinflammation. In this chapter, we summarise our current knowledge and existing gaps on post-injury NET formation.

2. Post-injury inflammation

2.1. Complications of post-injury inflammation

Major trauma patients universally develop systemic inflammatory response syndrome (SIRS) criteria within 72 h of injury. SIRS is defined by the following criteria:

a. Temperature greater than 38°C or less than 36°C.

b. Heart rate greater than 90 beats/min.

c. Respiratory rate greater than 20/min.

d. White blood cell count (WBC) greater than 12.0×10^9 L^{-1}, or less than 4.0×10^9 L^{-1} [6].

The degree of the dysfunctional post-injury inflammation is further complicated by the invasive nature of surgical procedures. Moreover, those who survive the initial severe tissue injury and traumatic shock are at an increased risk of acute respiratory distress syndrome (ARDS), multiple organ failure (MOF), nosocomial infections and sepsis. These complications lead to excessive resource utilisation and increased risk of death [7–9]. The systemic inflammatory response to major trauma can lead to the development of early MOF, which progresses to a state of immune paralysis and is viewed as a major factor underlying the increased susceptibility of trauma patients to hospital-acquired infections [10, 11]. The possible involvement of NETs in post-injury inflammation has been evaluated in several recent studies. Margraf and co-workers published in 2008 that NET quantities in plasma may predict MOF and sepsis on the ICU in patients after multiple trauma [12], and more recently, cell free-DNA neutrophil extracellular traps (cf-DNA/NETs) were used in the prediction of mortality in a population of 32 patients with severe burn injury [13]. These associations warrant further research into the precise role and impact of NETosis in the post-injury inflammatory response. While many aspects of the post-injury inflammatory response have been characterised over the past decades, our understanding of how NETosis fits into the picture is still rudimentary.

2.2. Mechanisms of post-injury inflammation

In the bigger picture of the post-injury inflammatory response, NETosis is considered a later phenomenon than the classical neutrophils functions [14–16]. Before the induction of NETosis, inflammatory reactions triggered by mechanical injury or disturbances of homeostasis are mainly propagated by intravascular events, summarised in **Figure 1**. The acute phase is characterised by dramatic changes in the diameter of the capillaries and the activation of innate immune cell responses. It is followed by a delayed, subacute reaction, most prominently characterised by oxido-reductive burst, hypoxic metabolic pathways, the infiltration of leukocytes and phagocytic cells and early cytokine production, while in the late proliferative phase, reperfusion injury, further production of late inflammatory agents, tissue remodelling and fibrosis occur.

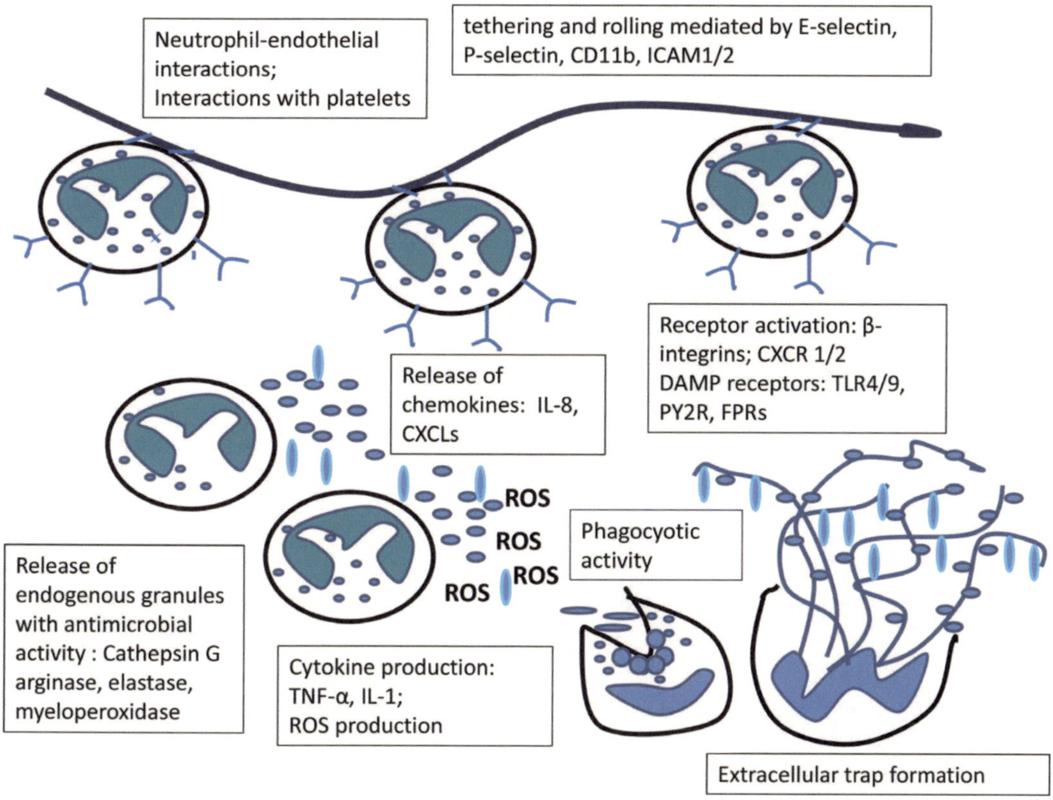

Figure 1. Schematic figure about multiple functions of neutrophils in response to sterile inflammation, where CD11b, integrin alpha M; ICAM, intercellular adhesion molecule; IL-8, interleukin-8 (chemokine receptor ligand 8); CXCLs, chemokine ligands; CXCR, chemokine receptor; DAMP, damage associated molecular pattern; TLR, Toll like receptor; IL-1, interleukin 1; PY2R, purinergic receptor; FPR, formyl peptide receptors; and TNFα, tumor necrosis factor-alpha.

Injury leads to the release of damage-associated molecular patterns (DAMPs) with high immunomodulatory potential (extracellular DNA, mitochondrial remnants and the high mobility group box 1) and pro-inflammatory cytokines, such as tumour necrosis factor-α (TNF-α), or interleukin-1β (IL-1β). Release of these components results in Toll-like receptor (TLR) activation with an effect after 1–2 h [17]. As this phase ensues, subacute cytokines including IL-6, IL-8 as well as IL-12 and IL-18, chemokines and leukocyte migratory factors drive an exaggerated activation of PMN leukocytes, and the increased production of reactive oxygen species (ROS) plays important roles in the process [18]. It is also widely accepted that the initial pro-inflammatory phase switches to a later anti-inflammatory phase with extended anti-inflammatory cytokine release to facilitate regenerative processes; however, the pro-inflammatory and anti-inflammatory forces may ultimately reinforce each other, creating a state of increasingly destructive immunologic dissonance [19]. Cytokine signals are crucial in the inflammatory cascade by promoting the interactions of PMN leukocytes with endothelial cells through the up-regulation of adhesion molecules, PMN degranulation, respiratory burst, lipid mediator synthesis [20] and enhanced migration through the endothelium. Via these reactions, the soluble mediators alter the microvascular homeostasis [21, 22] and blood flow, which have been associated with multiple organ failure [23]. Of the cytokines, members of the low molecular weight chemokine family play a fundamental part in these events by virtue of their ability to attract and stimulate leukocytes [24]. These mediators mutually and strictly regulate the expression level and generation of each via epigenetic regulation that propagate the commencement of repair mechanisms, although numerous cytokines are reported to be aberrantly regulated in association with more complicated clinical outcomes [25, 26].

While phagocytosis and degranulation usually take minutes to occur after being exposed to the inflammatory signal, NETosis is a more protracted event, takes place from 2–3 h up to 8 h from activation [27, 28]. About 20–60% of isolated human neutrophils typically release NETs 2–4 h after stimulation with microbes or chemicals [2]. However, they were able to respond within minutes when activated by LPS-stimulated platelets under conditions of flow [29]. These studies suggest that NET formation might be more characteristic for the subacute/late phase of post-injury inflammation and probably more inherent to the senescent PMN population. It is hoped that future studies will identify which factors determine the selection between these alternative antimicrobial activities and whether these processes can coexist in the same cell (**Figure 1**).

3. Mechanisms of NETosis

As members of the first-line defence of the immune system, neutrophils are well known to interact with other cell types and active cellular crosstalk is followed by release of inflammatory mediators, stimuli-specific receptor-activation and homing. NET formation is described to occur in a particularly versatile manner under different pathophysiological conditions, and the complexity is just the beginning to be explored. We are yet to clarify which factors are required to prevent NET formation of a neutrophil and whether this alternative pro-inflammatory function of the cells can co-exist with the classical responses of the same cell. The current view of the role of surrounding cells, soluble mediators and intracellular elements is overviewed below.

3.1. Structure and function of NETs

NETosis has been described as a process in which activated neutrophils extrude a chromatin-fibre-based meshwork encompassing their own granules and antimicrobial enzymes, such as neutrophil elastase, cathepsin G, α-defensines and MPO [1]. Mass spectrometry results have revealed a series of additional protein components from various types of granules [30]. The extrinsic and intrinsic factors contributing to NET formation are summarised in **Figure 2**.

These structures represent an important strategy to immobilise and kill invading microorganisms and are considered to be evolutionarily conserved, since they target both Gram-negative and Gram-positive bacteria, viruses and fungi [31]. Besides humans, the phenomenon

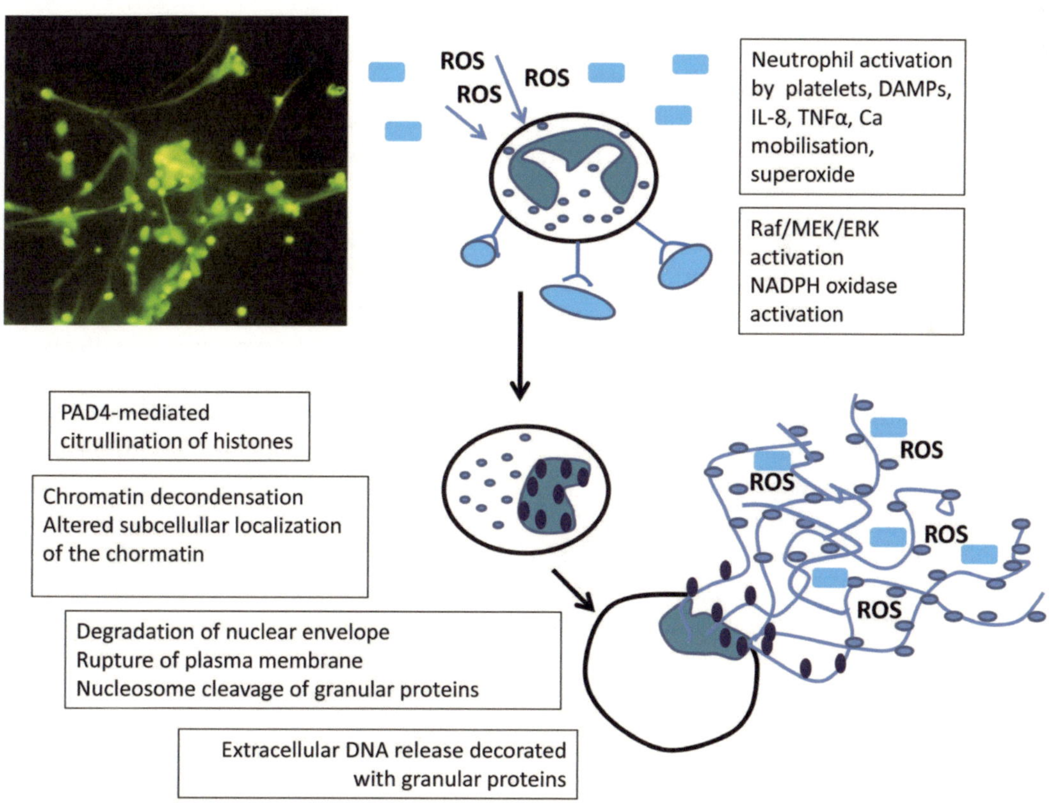

Figure 2. (A) Representative image of neutrophils forming extracellular traps visualized by fluorescent microscopy (Nikon Diaphot 300 Inverted fluorescence & phase contrast microscope, 20× magnification) after staining the cells with Sytox Green DNA intercalating dye. (B) Schematic figure on the possible mechanism of NET formation, where DAMP, damage-associated molecular pattern; IL-8, interleukin 8; TNFα, tumor necrosis factor-alpha; Raf, rapidly accelerated fibrosarcoma kinase; MEK, mitogen-activated protein kinase; ERK, extracellular signal regulated kinase; NADPH, nicotinamide adenine dinucleotide phosphate.and PAD4, protein arginine deiminase 4.

was proven to be present in insects, various vertebrates including fishes and even in plants [32–36]. The NET scaffold consists of chromatin components with a diameter of 15–17 nm and the connected proteins and microparticles. To date, nuclear DNA and histones are observed to represent the major NET constituents [1]. The exact mechanism through which the genetic material is ejected from the cell and decorated by antimicrobial factors is still not well understood. Nonetheless, it is considered to be an active process, where the cells undergo an apoptosis-like process with peptidylarginiedeamilase 4 (PAD-4)-mediated DNA decondensation, membrane disintegration and chromatin realignment [37], and the role of ROS formation in the process seems to be inevitable, but the mechanism remains controversial [2].

3.2. Post-injury activators of NETosis

Studies aimed at describing the receptor-ligand signalling pathways are fundamental in sterile NET formation revealed diverse and sometimes controversial mechanistic details. Endogenous ligands were described to bind to TLR (mainly TLR4 and TLR9), Fc receptors (e.g. FcRIIa) or cytokine receptors (such as IL-17 R) accompanied by this process [38–40]. Complement receptor activation has also been reported to be implicated [41]. Many sterile chemical stimuli were proven to induce NETosis *in vitro* without infection such as TNF-alpha, IL-8, interferon-gamma, nicotine certain antibiotics or enhanced ROS generation produced by NADPH oxidases [1, 42–46].

As NETs consist of a significant amount of extracellular DNA as a scaffold, injury-related NET formation may cause a further elevated DAMP concentration in the circulation, and therefore, it could result in more severe tissue damage [4, 48]. Mitochondrial DNA was subsequently demonstrated to be a trigger for NETosis after major trauma and demonstrated that the signalling was mediated through a TLR9-dependent pathway, independent of the NADPH oxidase system [39]. Our group demonstrated that NETs formed after trauma were almost exclusively composed of mtDNA [4]. There has also been a relationship demonstrated in NETosis observed in systemic lupus erythematous (SLE) where NETs released were found to be highly enriched with oxidised mtDNA [49]. Interestingly, this study also found that these NETs resulted in increased production of IFN I, which was dependent on STING pathway signalling. This perhaps suggests that mtDNA may play a role in driving autoimmunity in a rather novel and previously unstudied way.

3.3. Cell-cell interactions as regulators of post-injury NET formation

3.3.1. Interaction with platelets

There is growing evidence on the importance of neutrophil-neutrophil crosstalk and communication with other cells related to NET formation. Platelets are far the most characterised players in NETosis as many platelet originated ligand/receptor pairs and soluble mediators perpetuate neutrophil activation [50]. The proof-of-concept *in vitro* studies demonstrated that platelet activation is crucial as the initial step [29, 51]. Human neutrophils isolated from healthy volunteers underwent a robust NET formation in the presence of activated platelets treated with thrombin receptor-activating peptide, while no NETosis occurred with the co-incubation of resting platelets [52]. In the same study, the early event of platelet-platelet interaction was blocked with a glycoprotein IIb/IIIa inhibitor and resulted in reduced NET formation in a mice TRALI model [52]. P-selectin is suspected to largely be responsible for the ability to trigger sterile NET formation in human neutrophils [53], but other cell adhesion molecules found on platelets are demonstrated to play rather significant role as β2 integrin (CD18) [53, 54]. Among soluble mediators, chemokines (as CXCL4) and alarmins (as HMGB-1) produced by platelets were observed to activate neutrophils to form NETs *in vitro* and in animal models [54, 55]; however, this feature of platelets is broadly connected to any kind of inflammatory response, and therefore, the direct or indirect contribution of this phenomenon is too limited to be predictable.

3.3.2. Endothelium-neutrophil interactions

Circulating neutrophils tend to be quiescent and inactive, while their activation classically depends on their communication with endothelial cells. After neutrophil-endothelial interaction, the cells can rapidly undergo degranulation, activation of their NADPH oxidase system and even NET formation [56, 57]. The importance of this interface is also supported by more recent studies, where endothelium-produced matrix metalloproteinases induced NET formation followed by cytotoxicity and vessel dysfunction [58, 59].

3.4. Intracellular and molecular regulators of NETosis

Neutrophil extracellular trap formation is primarily dependent on histone abundance and alignment, activation of NADPH oxidase and MPO, interactions between platelets and neutrophils, expression of NET component proteins, and neutrophil autophagy.

3.4.1. The role of chromatin decondensation

Peptidylargininedeiminase 4 (PAD4)-mediated chromatin decondensation, which occurs in the nucleus, is apparently a critical and initial step in NET formation. PAD4 is a nuclear enzyme that converts specific arginine residues to citrulline on histone tails [60]. The release of NETs strongly depends on PAD4 activity [61] but was surprisingly found not to be essential in certain conditions [62]. Neutrophils isolated from PAD4-deficient mice were unable to citrullinate histones, decondense chromatin, and generate NETs [63]. In fact, PAD inhibitors have demonstrated efficacy in a variety of immune pathologies [64, 65], supporting the importance of this pathway in NET formation.

3.4.2. NADPH-dependent ROS production, Raf-MEK-ERK pathway

Hakkim and co-workers first described the importance of the Raf/MEK/ERK signalling pathway in PMA-induced NET formation and their data suggest that the Raf-MEK-ERK pathway might be upstream of NADPH oxidase activation [66]. Other studies pointed out that phosphorylation of ERK both in platelets and in neutrophils is also necessary for the formation of NETs mediated by activated platelets [52, 53].

3.4.3. Toll-like receptors

Toll-like receptors are classified according to the types of agonists that bind and the corresponding response that is activated and several of them were found to facilitate profound inflammatory responses after binding endogenous ligands [67]. It was recently reported that neutrophil stimulation via TLR activation with various molecules leads to NET production. Further to this, the structure of the NETs is characteristic to the type of TLR stimulation [68]. TLR4 seems to be responsible for this kind of neutrophil activity in particular as many publications demonstrated their interaction via HMGB-1 [55], superoxide production [69], platelet activation [29] or IL-1β [70]. Oxidised low-density lipoprotein, which has been implicated as an independent risk factor in various acute or chronic inflammatory diseases including SIRS, was also found to act as a NETosis trigger via TLRs [71]. More recently, TLR9 has come into focus in NET research as mtDNA and other DAMPs that are recognised by TLR9 showed high potential to induce NETs in trauma patients [39], in liver ischemia/reperfusion injury [3] or due to surgical stress [72].

4. Pathophysiology of post-injury NETs

4.1. The role of NETs in sterile inflammation

Recent discoveries have revealed the potential role of NETs in the pathogenesis of a wide range of non-infectious diseases, in particular sterile chronic inflammatory conditions such as systemic lupus erythematous [38, 73], small vessel vasculitis [74] and psoriasis [75]. In such conditions, both spontaneous NET formation and impaired NETosis were evident. Reduced ability of PMNs for to undergo NETosis was described in diabetes mellitus patients who were exposed to bacterial infections [76] that might be a possible explanation for why this population is more susceptible to life-threatening infections. In another recent study conducted on diabetes patients, spontaneous release of isolated PMN NETs was increased, suggesting that a chronic pro-inflammatory condition during hyperglycaemia favours constitutive NET formation [77]. Chronic inflammation is also characteristic in cardiovascular diseases and indeed, NETosis was found to contribute to the pathomechanism of deep vein thrombosis [78], acute myocardial ischemia/reperfusion in a mouse model [79], and NETs were observed to be localised in limb artherosclerotic plaques [80]. Furthermore, the content of plasma MPO-DNA complexes was found to be associated with an increased risk of coronary stenosis in patients with severe coronary arthelosclerosis [81]. Interestingly, healthy conditions but with an altered metabolic and oxygen consumption rate were also described to be associated with elevated NETosis of isolated PMNs. In a very recent paper, NET formation and neutrophil pro-NETotic priming were found to be augmented during the course pregnancy in healthy women when compared to matching non-pregnant control donors [82]. What was found to be elevated in the mother, seemed to be blocked in the foetus, as newborn neutrophils isolated from umbilical cord blood on the day of delivery did not form NETs when stimulated [83]. In the latter study, the authors identified a unique protein in the umbilical cord blood-called neonatal NET-inhibitory factor (nNIF) that would raise a very interesting question of a novel foetal adaptation mechanism and therapeutic approach. Acute injuries such as AKI and ALI were both described to be relevant pathologies to study increased NETosis in humans. NET biomarkers were present in transfusion-related acute lung injury patients' blood, and in fact, NETs were produced *in vitro* by primed human neutrophils when challenged with anti-neutrophil alloantigen-3a antibodies previously implicated in TRALI [84]. In another human study, the cfDNA/NET content of 31 critically ill patient's blood was in a significant positive correlation with the severity of acute kidney injury [85]. This result encouraged the evaluation of serum (or plasma) NETs concentration as an early predictive biomarkers of complicated outcomes on the ICU.

4.2. Pathophysiology of trauma-related NET formation

The potential role of NETs in the mechanical injury driven inflammatory response has recently been proposed [47, 86]. Similarly, the presence of NETs was demonstrated in a mixed intensive care unit population with systemic inflammatory response syndrome [87]. NETs have also been implicated in the pathogenesis of acute lung injury and in sterile transfusion-related acute lung injury, which are often antecedents of MOF [52]. Recently, Grimberg-Peters et al. published that neutrophils isolated from severely injured patients (days 1–2 after trauma) showed markedly elevated NET formation after pharmacological activation, and this effect was successfully attenuated by the treatment with hyperbaric oxygen [88]. This result indicates the potential importance of oxido-reductive burst in NETosis after traumatic injury, and it is well established that in such conditions, NET formation is generally NADPH oxidase-dependent [48]. However, the exact molecular mechanism behind is not fully understood, as indicated in a study by Itagakai and co-worker, where human PMNs from young and elderly trauma patients formed NETs in a great number, via TLR9 activation, but independently from NADPH oxidase activation [39].

Moreover, the DAMP release after trauma might be fundamental in further promoting NET production. Besides its role in sterile inflammation, mitochondrial DNA may have another pivotal role in worsening the inflammatory response, via NET formation. Our recent data show NETs observed after injury and subsequent surgery can be composed of mitochondrial DNA [4], and other authors have found the same phenomenon under certain conditions [89]. The exact molecular mechanism of mtDNA-NET release is unclear; however, when a ROS production inhibitor (diphenyleneiodonium) was used, mitochondrial DNA-NET formation was also blocked, and no DNA was released [89, 90].

4.3. NETs as therapeutic target for post-injury inflammation

To date, the contribution of NET formation on the pathomechanism of a wide range of clinical conditions is evident, and there is emerging evidence about the potential therapeutic usefulness of pharmacological NET inhibition. While animal experiments and *in vitro* cell culture studies are promising, it is yet unknown if NET-targeting therapies can be effective in clinical practice. As many protective physiological and pathophysiological processes require NET formation, the harm/benefit ratio of NET formation inhibition is unclear.

4.3.1. Chemical inhibition of NETosis

There are several drugs already used in clinical practice in autoimmune diseases that have potential for NETosis inhibition. Plaquenil Sulphate (hydroxychloroquine, HQ) is a disease-modifying anti-rheumatic drug, which inhibits prostaglandin and cytokine synthesis, and most of all induces a blockade in TLR signalling [91]. Juvenile-onset systemic lupus erythematosus patients' isolated PMNs showed augmented NET formation, which was significantly modulated with HQ treatment [92]. N-acetylcisteine (NAC), which is a commonly recommended supplement to treat various autoimmune symptoms, was described to inhibit NET release by PMA stimulated human neutrophils in a ROS-dependent manner [93]. The application of NAC had similar effect in other recently published studies [70, 94], which supports the usage of other free radical scavengers as adjuvant therapy on the ICU trauma patients. Monoclonal antibodies such as the complement inhibitor Eculizumab might open up a new perspective in drug therapies targeting NETosis based on the findings that plasma NET markers of paroxysmal nocturnal haemoglobinuria patients with thrombosis history were significantly elevated than that of controls or patients without thrombosis history, while the Eculizumab treatment normalised the values to the control level [95]. Another FDA-approved monoclonal antibody, Rituximab was also demonstrated to be protective against adverse NET formation in different human studies [96].

The inhibition of histone decondensation via PAD4 targeting of the PMNs is another potential NET-based therapeutic target, as PAD overexpression and upregulated enzyme activity have been observed in several diseases [97], and or PAD4-mediated NET formation was described to be not essential against infection [62].

The direct inhibition of the granule and protein components of NETs is another way to manipulate NET formation. However, these are essential antimicrobial peptides and mediate important physiological pathways. Currently, the literature is conflicting as to whether MPO, NE and the other compounds connected to the NET scaffold are appropriate targets. In one study, MPO-facilitated ROS-generation was proven to be required for neutrophil extracellular trap formation in humans and pharmacological inhibition of MPO delays and reduces NET formation [28, 98, 99], but recently more evidence revealed the opposite or conditional effect [100–102].

4.3.2. The therapeutic effect of DNAse treatment

The fact that extrachromosomal DNA and particularly mtDNA have such potent immunostimulatory effects makes it an exciting and very rational target for immunomodulation therapy and silencing NET formation is one of the many possible trends. Whether nDNA or mtDNA are conjugated with NETs, both are readily digestible with DNAse. There is certainly good evidence to suggest that focally targeting NETs with DNAse have yielded a reduction in associated inflammatory lung damage in a mouse model of transfusion-related acute lung injury (TRALI) [52]. Human recombinant DNAse therapy has been used to good effect when nebulised in cystic fibrosis (CF) patients by enhancing sputum solubilisation [103]. This effect may be beneficial to other conditions with excessive NETosis, as several studies have recently demonstrated that NETs and NET-associated proteins are present in CF sputum [104–107].

However, there might be dangerous consequences if the extracellular DNA is not cleared up perfectly or if the freely floating pro-inflammatory peptides have entered the bloodstream. Dubois and colleagues have demonstrated that DNase administration to CF sputum dramatically increased elastase activity [108]. Thus, the combined administration of DNase and specific inhibitor could be useful to avoid the deleterious effects of excessive proteases. With such an emergent role of mtDNA in NETs associated with trauma [4] and more recently in SLE [49], the investigation of DNAse therapy in different inflammatory conditions including post-injury inflammation would be very reasonable. Nevertheless, a long-term DNase therapy presents side effects to patients [109] including dramatic increase in other antimicrobial activities [108] or further impedance of the immune system which makes the host susceptible to disseminated and lethal infections [110, 111]. The latter has notable consideration in the management of major trauma patient as 39.5% of trauma deaths occur in the hospital mainly due to nosocomial infections [112].

4.3.3. *The clinical predictive value of NETs*

The number of studies investigating the presence or the predictive value of NETs and NET components alongside extracellular DNA concentration as potential biomarkers in different human body fluids has grown significantly in recent years. Serum and plasma certainly are the most investigated materials, as being the natural habitat for PMNs, although it raises some concern whether activated NET-forming PMNs are representative enough in the blood.

In cases of acute injuries, such as major trauma, quantification of NETs from blood seems to be a trustworthy biomarker for clinical prediction. Margraf and co-workers published in 2008 that NETs quantities in plasma may predict multiple organ failure and sepsis on the ICU in patients after multiple trauma [12]. This ground breaking work was followed by other papers, such as the one of Altrichter and co-workers who described that circulating free-DNA neutrophil extracellular traps (cf-DNA/NETs) could be used in the prediction of mortality in a population of 32 patients with severe burn injury [13]. Similarly, early diagnosis of septic arthritis by cfDNA/NETs measurement could guide the surgical team to rescue the joint by deciding to perform an immediate operation [99]. However, in these cases, the dynamic profile of circulating neutrophils and NETs in the acute and subacute phase of inflammation should be taken into consideration when determining the optimal timing of biomarker measurement. It is also important to note that NET components, namely DNA complexes and elastase, may also accumulate in the blood during other programs of cell death, for example, during endothelial cell apoptosis or macrophage necrosis [81].

Beyond blood-based extracellular trap identification, Mohanty and co-workers described a new approach to non-invasive NET-associated biomarker research, which showed the presence of numerous neutrophils in morning saliva had undergone NETosis [113]. Tear fluid might also be informative. In a study conducted on dry eye disease (DED) patients and matching controls, tear fluid nuclease activity was decreased significantly in DED patients, whereas the amount of extracellular DNA, histones, cathelicidin, and neutrophil elastase on the ocular surface was increased significantly [114]. A similar paper characterised the activated neutrophil-specific biomarkers in the tear fluid among ocular graft versus host disease patients, and a marked increase in both NE and MPO concentrations was evident [115].

5. Final remarks

In this chapter, we summarised the mechanism, regulation and clinical significance of neutrophil granulocytes and the complex process of extracellular trap formation. The relevant literature shows that a highly specialised population of neutrophils facilitate NET formation in response to infection and also sterile inflammation. Interest in the potential role of NETs in the posttraumatic injury setting and their possible role in the subsequent inflammatory response has gained significant attention lately. To date, the contribution of NET formation on the pathomechanism of a wide range of clinical conditions was proven to be inevitable and the observation of NETosis became more important in post-injury clinical outcome prediction.

For the better understanding of the exact mechanistic details and the role of NETs in normal recovery and disease, improved methodology and quantification are urgently needed. The current techniques combine fluorescent microscopy or fluorescent intensity measurements and generally use DNA-intercalating dyes, while taking the risk of visualising necrotic cells with dye permeable cell membrane. Antibody-based techniques are required to detect activated, non-necrotic cells with intact cell membrane, such as flow cytometry-cell-sorting, supported by microscopic imaging. Additionally, a consensus on the structural and behavioural definition of NET formation is essential for future NET research, due to their fragility, their highly dynamic nature and their morphological heterogeneity.

Author details

Eszter Tuboly[1], Gabrielle D. Briggs[2] and Zsolt J. Balogh[1,2]*

*Address all correspondence to: zsolt.balogh@hnehealth.nsw.gov.au

1 Hunter New England Health, Newcastle, Australia

2 University of Newcastle, Newcastle, Australia

References

[1] Brinkmann V, Reichard U, Goosmann C, Fauler B, Uhlemann Y, Weiss DS, Weinrauch Y, Zychlinsky A. Neutrophil extracellular traps kill bacteria. Science. 2004 Mar;**303**(5663):1532–1535

[2] Kaplan MJ, Radic M. Neutrophil extracellular traps: Double-edged swords of innate immunity. The Journal of Immunology. 2012 Sep;**189**(6):2689–2695

[3] Huang HS, Tohme S, Al-Khafaji AB, Tai S, Loughran P, Chen L, Wang S, Kim J, Billiar T, Wang Y, Tsung A. Damage-associated molecular pattern-activated neutrophil extracellular trap exacerbates sterile inflammatory liver injury. Hepatology. 2015 Aug;**62**(2):600–614

[4] McIlroy DJ, Jarnicki AG, Au GG, Lott N, Smith DW, Hansbro PM, Balogh ZJ. Mitochondrial DNA neutrophil extracellular traps are formed after trauma and subsequent surgery. Journal of Critical Care. 2014 Dec;**29**(6):1133.e1–e5

[5] Leliefeld PH, Wessels CM, Leenen LP, Koenderman L, Pillay J. The role of neutrophils in immune dysfunction during severe inflammation. Critical Care. 2016 Mar;**20**:73

[6] Klein Klouwenberg PM, Ong DS, Bonten MJ, Cremer OL. Classification of sepsis, severe sepsis and septic shock: The impact of minor variations in data capture and definition of SIRS criteria. Intensive Care Medicine. 2012 May;**38**(5):811–819

[7] Osborn TM, Tracy JK, Dunne JR, Pasquale M, Napolitano LM. Epidemiology of sepsis in patients with traumatic injury. Critical Care Medicine. 2004 Nov;**32**(11):2234–2240

[8] Lazarus HM, Fox J, Burke JP, Lloyd JF, Snow GL, Mehta RR, Evans RS, Abouzelof R, Taylor C, Stevens MH. Trauma patient hospital-associated infections: Risks and outcomes. Journal of Trauma and Acute Care Surgery. 2005 Jul;**59**(1):188–194

[9] Gutierrez T, Hornigold R, Pearce A. The systemic response to surgery. Surgery. 2014 March;**32**(3):149–152

[10] Glance LG, Stone PW, Mukamel DB, Dick AW. Increases in mortality, length of stay, and cost associated with hospital-acquired infections in trauma patients. The Art and Science of Surgery. 2011 Jul;**146**(7):794–801

[11] Hietbrink F, Koenderman L, Rijkers G, Leenen L. Trauma: The role of the innate immune system. World Journal of Emergency Surgery. 2006 May **20**;1:15

[12] Dewar D, Moore FA, Moore EE, Balogh Z. Postinjury multiple organ failure. Injury. 2009 Sep;**40**(9):912–918

[13] Margraf S, Lögters T, Reipen J, Altrichter J, Scholz M, Windolf J. Neutrophil-derived circulating free DNA (cf-DNA/NETs): A potential prognostic marker for posttraumatic development of inflammatory second hit and sepsis. Shock. 2008 Oct;**30**(4):352–358

[14] Altrichter J, Zedler S, Kraft R, Faist E, Mitzner SR, Sauer M, Windolf J, Scholz M, Lögters T. Neutrophil-derived circulating free DNA (cf-DNA/NETs), a potential prognostic marker for mortality in patients with severe burn injury. European Journal of Trauma and Emergency Surgery. 2010 Dec;**36**(6):551–557

[15] Brinkmann V, Zychlinsky A. Neutrophil extracellular traps: Is immunity the second function of chromatin? The Journal of Cell Biology. 2012 Sep;**198**(5):773–783

[16] Tibrewal S, Ivanir Y, Sarkar J, Nayeb-Hashemi N, Bouchard CS, Kim E, Jain S. Hyperosmolar stress induces neutrophil extracellular trap formation: Implications for dry eye disease. Investigative Ophthalmology & Visual Science. 2014 Nov;**55**(12):7961–7969

[17] Helseth R, Solheim S, Arnesen H, Seljeflot I, Opstad TB. The time course of markers of neutrophil extracellular traps in patients undergoing revascularization for acute myocardial infarction or stable angina pectoris. Mediators of Inflammation. 2016;**2016**:2182358

[18] Keel M, Trentz O. Pathophysiology of polytrauma. Injury. 2005 Jun;**36**(6):691–709

[19] Ward PA, Lentsch AB. The acute inflammatory response and its regulation. Archives of Surgery. 1999 Jun;**134**(6):666–669

[20] Bone RC. Immunologic dissonance: A continuing evolution in our understanding of the systemic inflammatory response syndrome (SIRS) and the multiple organ dysfunction syndrome (MODS). Annals of Internal Medicine. 1996 Oct;**125**(8):680–687

[21] Baggiolini M, Dewald B, Moser B. Interleukin-8 and related chemotactic cytokines—CXC and CC chemokines. Advances in Immunology. 1994;**55**:97–179

[22] Dinarello CA. Role of pro- and anti-inflammatory cytokines during inflammation: Experimental and clinical findings. Journal of Biological Regulators & Homeostatic Agents. 1997 Jul-Sep;**11**(3):91–103

[23] Feghali CA, Wright TM. Cytokines in acute and chronic inflammation. Frontiers in Bioscience. 1997 Jan;**2**:d12–d26

[24] Trzeciak S, Dellinger RP, Parrillo JE, Guglielmi M, Bajaj J, Abate NL, Arnold RC, Colilla S, Zanotti S, Hollenberg SM. Microcirculatory alterations in resuscitation and shock investigators. Annals of Emergency Medicine. 2007 Jan;**49**(1):88–98, 98.e1–e2

[25] Kunkel SL, Strieter RM, Lindley IJ, Westwick J. Chemokines: New ligands, receptors and activities. Immunology Today. 1995 Dec;**16**(12):559–561

[26] Wen H, Dou Y, Hogaboam CM, Kunkel SL. Epigenetic regulation of dendritic cell-derived interleukin-12 facilitates immunosuppression after a severe innate immune response. Blood. 2008 Feb;**111**(4):1797–1804

[27] Bataille A, Galichon P, Ziliotis MJ, Sadia I, Hertig A. Epigenetic changes during sepsis: On your marks! Critical Care. 2015 Oct;**19**:358

[28] Brinkmann V, Laube B, Abu Abed U, Goosmann C, Zychlinsky A. Neutrophil extracellular traps: How to generate and visualize them. Journal of Visualized Experiments. 2010 Feb;(**36**):1724

[29] Metzler KD, Fuchs TA, Nauseef WM, Reumaux D, Roesler J, Schulze I, Wahn V, Papayannopoulos V, Zychlinsky A. Myeloperoxidase is required for neutrophil extracellular trap formation: Implications for innate immunity. Blood. 2011 Jan;**117**(3):953–959

[30] Clark SR, Ma AC, Tavener SA, McDonald B, Goodarzi Z, Kelly MM, Patel KD, Chakrabarti S, McAvoy E, Sinclair GD, Keys EM, Allen-Vercoe E, Devinney R, Doig CJ, Green FH, Kubes P. Platelet TLR4 activates neutrophil extracellular traps to ensnare bacteria in septic blood. Nature Medicine. 2007 Apr;**13**(4):463–469

[31] Jaillon S, Peri G, Delneste Y, Frémaux I, Doni A, Moalli F, Garlanda C, Romani L, Gascan H, Bellocchio S, Bozza S, Cassatella MA, Jeannin P, Mantovani A. The humoral pattern recognition receptor PTX3 is stored in neutrophil granules and localizes in extracellular traps. The Journal of Experimental Medicine. 2007 Apr;**204**(4):793–804

[32] Urban CF, Lourido S, Zychlinsky A. How do microbes evade neutrophil killing? Cellular Microbiology. 2006 Nov;**8**(11):1687–1696

[33] Palić D, Ostojić J, Andreasen CB, Roth JA. Fish cast NETs: Neutrophil extracellular traps are released from fish neutrophils. Developmental & Comparative Immunology. 2007;**31**(8):805–816

[34] Altincicek B, Stötzel S, Wygrecka M, Preissner KT, Vilcinskas A. Host-derived extracellular nucleic acids enhance innate immune responses, induce coagulation, and prolong survival upon infection in insects. The Journal of Immunology. 2008 Aug;**181**(4):2705–2712

[35] Ermert D1, Urban CF, Laube B, Goosmann C, Zychlinsky A, Brinkmann V. Mouse neutrophil extracellular traps in microbial infections. Journal of Innate Immunity. 2009;**1**(3):181–193

[36] Wen F, White GJ, VanEtten HD, Xiong Z, Hawes MC. Extracellular DNA is required for root tip resistance to fungal infection. Plant Physiology. 2009 Oct;**151**(2):820–829

[37] Wardini AB, Guimarães-Costa AB, Nascimento MT, Nadaes NR, Danelli MG, Mazur C, Benjamim CF, Saraiva EM, Pinto-da-Silva LH. Characterization of neutrophil extracellular traps in cats naturally infected with feline leukemia virus. Journal of General Virology. 2010 Jan;**91**(Pt 1):259–264

[38] Fuchs TA, Abed U, Goosmann C, Hurwitz R, Schulze I, Wahn V, Weinrauch Y, Brinkmann V, Zychlinsky A. Novel cell death program leads to neutrophil extracellular traps. Journal of Cell Biology. 2007 Jan;**176**(2):231–241

[39] Garcia-Romo GS, Caielli S, Vega B, Connolly J, Allantaz F, Xu Z, Punaro M, Baisch J, Guiducci C, Coffman RL, Barrat FJ, Banchereau J, Pascual V. Netting neutrophils are major inducers of type I IFN production in pediatric systemic lupus erythematosus. Science Translational Medicine. 2011 Mar;**3**(73):73ra20

[40] Itagaki K, Kaczmarek E, Lee YT, Tang IT, Isal B, Adibnia Y, Sandler N, Grimm MJ, Segal BH, Otterbein LE, Hauser CJ. Mitochondrial DNA released by trauma induces neutrophil extracellular traps. PLoS One. 2015 Mar;**10**(3):e0120549

[41] Suzuki E, Maverakis E, Sarin R, Bouchareychas L, Kuchroo VK, Nestle FO. Adamopoulos IE. T Cell-independent mechanisms associated with neutrophil extracellular trap formation and selective autophagy in IL-17A-mediated epidermal hyperplasia. The Journal of Immunology. 2016 Dec;**197**(11):4403–4412

[42] Munks MW, McKee AS, Macleod MK, Powell RL, Degen JL, Reisdorph NA, Kappler JW, Marrack P. Aluminum adjuvants elicit fibrin-dependent extracellular traps in vivo. Blood. 2010 Dec;**116**(24):5191–5199

[43] Keshari RS, Jyoti A, Dubey M, Kothari N, Kohli M, Bogra J, Barthwal MK, Dikshit M. Cytokines induced neutrophil extracellular traps formation: Implication for the inflammatory disease condition. PLoS One. 2012;**7**(10):e48111

[44] Björnsdottir H1, Granfeldt D, Welin A, Bylund J, Karlsson A. Inhibition of phospholipase A(2) abrogates intracellular processing of NADPH-oxidase derived reactive oxygen species in human neutrophils. Experimental Cell Research. 2013 Mar;**319**(5):761–774

[45] Zawrotniak M, Rapala-Kozik M. Neutrophil extracellular traps (NETs)—Formation and implications. Acta Biochimica Polonica. 2013;**60**(3):277–884

[46] Hosseinzadeh A, Thompson PR, Segal BH, Urban CF. Nicotine induces neutrophil extracellular traps. Journal of Leukocyte Biology. 2016 Nov;**100**(5):1105–1112

[47] Manda-Handzlik A, Bystrzycka W, Sieczkowska S, Demkow U, Ciepiela O. Antibiotics modulate the ability of neutrophils to release neutrophil extracellular traps. Advances in Experimental Medicine and Biology. 20 Sep 2016. [Epub ahead of print]

[48] Liu FC, Chuang YH, Tsai YF, Yu HP. Role of neutrophil extracellular traps following injury. Shock. 2014 Jun;**41**(6):491–498

[49] Almyroudis NG, Grimm MJ, Davidson BA, Röhm M, Urban CF, Segal BH. NETosis and NADPH oxidase: At the intersection of host defense, inflammation, and injury. Frontiers in Immunology. 2013 Mar;**4**:45

[50] Lood C, Blanco LP, Purmalek MM, Carmona-Rivera C, De Ravin SS, Smith CK, Malech HL, Ledbetter JA, Elkon KB, Kaplan MJ. Neutrophil extracellular traps enriched in oxidized mitochondrial DNA are interferogenic and contribute to lupus-like disease. Nature Medicine. 2016 Feb;**22**(2):146–153

[51] Kazzaz NM, Sule G, Knight JS. Intercellular interactions as regulators of NETosis. Frontiers in Immunology. 2016;**7**:453. eCollection 2016

[52] Maugeri N, Campana L, Gavina M, Covino C, De Metrio M, Panciroli C, Maiuri L, Maseri A, D'Angelo A, Bianchi ME, Rovere-Querini P, ManfrediAA. Activated platelets present high mobility group box 1 to neutrophils, inducing autophagy and promoting the extrusion of neutrophil extracellular traps. Journal of Thrombosis and Haemostasis. 2014 Dec;**12**(12):2074–2088

[53] Caudrillier A, Kessenbrock K, Gilliss BM, Nguyen JX, Marques MB, Monestier M, Toy P, Werb Z, Looney MR. Platelets induce neutrophil extracellular traps in transfusion-related acute lung injury. Journal of Clinical Investigation. 2012 Jul;**122**(7):2661–2671

[54] Carestia A, Kaufman T, Schattner M. Platelets: New bricks in the building of neutrophil extracellular traps. Frontiers in Immunology. 2016 Jul;**7**:271

[55] Rossaint J, Herter JM, Van Aken H, Napirei M, Döring Y, Weber C, Soehnlein O, Zarbock A. Synchronized integrin engagement and chemokine activation is crucial in neutrophil extracellular trap-mediated sterile inflammation. Blood. 2014 Apr;**123**(16):2573–2584

[56] Tadie JM, Bae HB, Jiang S, Park DW, Bell CP, Yang H, Pittet JF, Tracey K, Thannickal VJ, Abraham E, Zmijewski JW. HMGB1 promotes neutrophil extracellular trap formation through interactions with Toll-like receptor 4. American Journal of Physiology. 2013 Mar;**304**(5):L342-L349

[57] Guthrie LA, McPhail LC, Henson PM, Johnston RB Jr. Priming of neutrophils for enhanced release of oxygen metabolites by bacterial lipopolysaccharide. Evidence for increased activity of the superoxide-producing enzyme. The Journal of Experimental Medicine. 1984 Dec;**160**(6):1656–1671

[58] Williams MR, Azcutia V, Newton G, Alcaide P, Luscinskas FW. Emerging mechanisms of neutrophil recruitment across endothelium. Trends in Immunology. 2011 Oct;**32**(10):461–469

[59] Gupta AK, Joshi MB, Philippova M, Erne P, Hasler P, Hahn S, Resink TJ. Activated endothelial cells induce neutrophil extracellular traps and are susceptible to NETosis-mediated cell death. FEBS Letters. 2010 Jul;**584**(14):3193–3197

[60] Saffarzadeh M, Juenemann C, Queisser MA, Lochnit G, Barreto G, Galuska SP, Lohmeyer J, Preissner KT. Neutrophil extracellular traps directly induce epithelial and endothelial cell death: A predominant role of histones. PLoS One. 2012;**7**(2):e32366

[61] Arita K, Shimizu T, Hashimoto H, Hidaka Y, Yamada M, Sato M. Structural basis for histone N-terminal recognition by human peptidylargininedeiminase 4. Proceedings of the National Academy of Sciences. 2006 Apr;**103**(14):5291–5296

[62] Rohrbach AS, Slade DJ, Thompson PR, Mowen KA. Activation of PAD4 in NET formation. Frontiers in Immunology. 2012 Nov ;**3**:360

[63] Hemmers S, Teijaro JR, Arandjelovic S, Mowen KA. PAD4-mediated neutrophil extracellular trap formation is not required for immunity against influenza infection. PLoS One. 2011;**6**(7):e22043

[64] Li P, Li M, Lindberg MR, Kennett MJ, Xiong N, Wang Y. PAD4 is essential for antibacterial innate immunity mediated by neutrophil extracellular traps. Journal of Experimental Medicine. 2010 Aug;**207**(9):1853–1862

[65] Chumanevich AA1, Causey CP, Knuckley BA, Jones JE, Poudyal D, Chumanevich AP, Davis T, Matesic LE, Thompson PR, Hofseth LJ. Suppression of colitis in mice by Cl-amidine: A novel peptidylargininedeiminase inhibitor. American Journal of Physiology. Gastrointestinal and Liver Physiology. 2011 Jun;**300**(6):G929–G938

[66] Willis VC, Gizinski AM, Banda NK, Causey CP, Knuckley B, Cordova KN, Luo Y, Levitt B, Glogowska M, Chandra P, Kulik L, Robinson WH, Arend WP, Thompson PR, Holers VM. N-α-benzoyl-N5-(2-chloro-1-iminoethyl)-L-ornithine amide, a protein arginine deiminase inhibitor, reduces the severity of murine collagen-induced arthritis. The Journal of Immunology. 2011 Apr;**186**(7):4396–4404

[67] Hakkim A, Fuchs TA, Martinez NE, Hess S, Prinz H, Zychlinsky A, Waldmann H. Activation of the Raf-MEK-ERK pathway is required for neutrophil extracellular trap formation. Nature Chemical Biology. 2011 Feb;**7**(2):75–77

[68] Holloway TL, Nicholson SE, Rani M, Cap AP, Schwacha MG. Toll-like receptor responses are suppressed in trauma ICU patients. Journal of Surgical Research. 2016 Nov;**206**(1):139–145

[69] Singh RR,RandhawaD, Valera I. Human neutrophil extracellular trap formation is modulated upon stimulation with Toll-like-receptor ligands. The Journal of Immunology. 2016 May;**196** (1 Supplement): 60.7

[70] Al-Khafaji AB, Tohme S, Yazdani HO, Miller D, Huang H, Tsung A. Superoxide induces neutrophil extracellular trap formation in a TLR-4 and NOX-dependent mechanism. Molecular Medicine. 2016 Jul;**22**:621–631

[71] Tashiro M, Sasatomi Y, Watanabe R, Watanabe M, Miyake K, Abe Y, Yasuno T, Ito K, Ueki N, Hamauchi A, Noda R, Hisano S, Nakashima H. IL-1β promotes tubulointerstitial injury in MPO-ANCA-associated glomerulonephritis. Clinical Nephrology. 2016 Oct;**86**(10):190–199

[72] Awasthi D, Nagarkoti S, Kumar A, Dubey M, Singh AK, Pathak P, Chandra T, Barthwal MK, Dikshit M. Oxidized LDL induced extracellular trap formation in human neutrophils via TLR-PKC-IRAK-MAPK and NADPH-oxidase activation. Free Radical Biology & Medicine. 2016 Apr;**93**:190–203

[73] Tohme S, Yazdani HO, Al-Khafaji AB, Chidi AP, Loughran P, Mowen K, Wang Y, Simmons RL, Huang H, Tsung A. Neutrophil extracellular traps promote the development and progression of liver metastases after surgical stress. Cancer Research. 2016 Mar;**76**(6):1367–1380

[74] Villanueva E, Yalavarthi S, Berthier CC, Hodgin JB, Khandpur R, Lin AM, Rubin CJ, Zhao W, Olsen SH, Klinker M, Shealy D, Denny MF, Plumas J, Chaperot L, Kretzler M, Bruce AT, Kaplan MJ. Netting neutrophils induce endothelial damage, infiltrate tissues, and expose immunostimulatorymolecules in systemic lupus erythematosus. The Journal of Immunology. 2011 Jul;**187**(1):538–552

[75] Nakazawa D, Tomaru U, Suzuki A, Masuda S, Hasegawa R, Kobayashi T, Nishio S, Kasahara M, Ishizu A. Abnormal conformation and impaired degradation of propylthiouracil-induced neutrophil extracellular traps: Implications of disordered neutrophil extracellular traps in a rat model of myeloperoxidase antineutrophil cytoplasmic antibody-associated vasculitis. Arthritis & Rheumatology. 2012 Nov;**64**(11):3779–3787

[76] Lin AM, Rubin CJ, Khandpur R, Wang JY, Riblett M, Yalavarthi S, Villanueva EC, Shah P, Kaplan MJ, Bruce AT. Mast cells and neutrophils release IL-17 through extracellular trap formation in psoriasis. The Journal of Immunology. 2011 Jul;**187**(1):490–500

[77] Riyapa D, Buddhisa S, Korbsrisate S, Cuccui J, Wren BW, Stevens MP, Ato M, Lertmemongkolchai G. Neutrophil extracellular traps exhibit antibacterial activity against burkholderia pseudomallei and are influenced by bacterial and host factors. Infection and Immunity. 2012 Nov;**80**(11):3921–3929

[78] Joshi MB, Lad A, Bharath Prasad AS, Balakrishnan A, Ramachandra L, Satyamoorthy K. High glucose modulates IL-6 mediated immune homeostasis through impeding neutrophil extracellular trap formation. FEBS Letters. 2013 Jul;**587**(14):2241–2246

[79] Fuchs TA, Brill A, Wagner DD. Neutrophil extracellular trap (NET) impact on deep vein thrombosis. Arteriosclerosis, Thrombosis, and Vascular Biology. 2012 Aug;**32**(8):1777–1783

[80] Savchenko AS, Borissoff JI, Martinod K, De Meyer SF, Gallant M, Erpenbeck L, Brill A, Wang Y, Wagner DD. VWF-mediated leukocyte recruitment with chromatin decondensation by PAD4 increases myocardial ischemia/reperfusion injury in mice. Blood. 2014 Jan;**123**(1):141–148

[81] Quillard T, Araújo HA, Franck G, Shvartz E, Sukhova G, Libby P. TLR2 and neutrophils potentiate endothelial stress, apoptosis and detachment: Implications for superficial erosion. European Heart Journal. 2015 Jun;**36**(22):1394–1404.

[82] Döring Y, Weber C, Soehnlein O. Footprints of neutrophil extracellular traps as predictors of cardiovascular risk. Arteriosclerosis, Thrombosis, and Vascular Biology. 2013 Aug;**33**(8):1735–1736

[83] Giaglis S, Stoikou M, Sur Chowdhury C, Schaefer G, Grimolizzi F, Rossi SW, Hoesli IM, Lapaire O, Hasler P, Hahn S. Multimodal regulation of NET formation in pregnancy: Progesterone antagonizes the Pro-NETotic effect of estrogen and G-CSF. Frontiers in Immunology. 2016 Dec;**7**:565

[84] Yost CC, Schwertz H, Cody MJ, Wallace JA, Campbell RA, Vieira-de-Abreu A, Araujo CV, Schubert S, Harris ES, Rowley JW, Rondina MT, Fulcher JM, Koening CL, Weyrich AS, Zimmerman GA. Neonatal NET-inhibitory factor and related peptides inhibit neutrophil extracellular trap formation. Journal of Clinical Investigation. 2016 Oct;**126**(10):3783–3798

[85] Thomas GM, Carbo C, Curtis BR, Martinod K, Mazo IB, Schatzberg D, Cifuni SM, Fuchs TA, von Andrian UH, Hartwig JH, Aster RH, Wagner DD. Extracellular DNA traps are associated with the pathogenesis of TRALI in humans and mice. Blood. 2012 Jun;**119**(26):6335–6343

[86] Czaikoski PG, Mota JM, Nascimento DC, Sônego F, Castanheira FV, Melo PH, Scortegagna GT, Silva RL, Barroso-Sousa R, Souto FO, Pazin-Filho A, Figueiredo F, Alves-Filho JC, Cunha FQ, Balogh ZJ, McIlroy DJ, Smith DW, Hansbro PM. The origin and the role of mitochondrial DNA in postinjury inflammation. Journal of Critical Care. 2013 Dec;**28**(6):1099–1100

[87] Hamaguchi S, Hirose T, Akeda Y, Matsumoto N, Irisawa T, Seki M, Hosotsubo H, Tasaki O, Oishi K, Shimazu T, Tomono K. Identification of neutrophil extracellular traps in the blood of patients with systemic inflammatory response syndrome. Journal of International Medical Research. 2013 Feb;**41**(1):162–168

[88] Grimberg-Peters D, Büren C, Windolf J, Wahlers T, Paunel-Görgülü A. Hyperbaric oxygen reduces production of reactive oxygen species in neutrophils from polytraumatized-patients yielding in the inhibition of p38 MAP Kinase and downstream pathways. PLoS One. 2016 Aug;**11**(8):e0161343

[89] Yousefi S, Mihalache C, Kozlowski E, Schmid I, Simon HU. Viable neutrophils release mitochondrial DNA to form neutrophil extracellular traps. Cell Death & Differentiation. 2009 Nov;**16**(11):1438–1444

[90] Yousefi S, Simon D, Simon HU. Eosinophil extracellular DNA traps: Molecular mechanisms and potential roles in disease. Current Opinion in Immunology. 2012 Dec;**24**(6):736–739

[91] Lee SJ, Silverman E, Bargman JM. The role of antimalarial agents in the treatment of SLE and lupus nephritis. Nature Reviews Nephrology. 2011 Oct;**7**(12):718–729

[92] Makuloluwa KK, Midgley A, Beresford M. Neutrophil extracellular trap-mediated activation of endosomal toll-like receptors induce immune activation in juvenile-onset systemic lupus erythematosus. Pediatric Rheumatology. 2014;**12**(Suppl 1):P110

[93] Kirchner T, Hermann E, Möller S, Klinger M, Solbach W, Laskay T, Behnen M. Flavonoids and 5-aminosalicylic acid inhibit the formation of neutrophil extracellular traps. Mediators of Inflammation. 2013;**2013**:710239

[94] Rada B, Jendrysik MA, Pang L, Hayes CP, Yoo DG, Park JJ, Moskowitz SM, Malech HL, Leto TL. Pyocyanin-enhanced neutrophil extracellular trap formation requires the NADPH oxidase. PLoS One. 2013;**8**(1):e54205

[95] vanBijnen ST, Wouters D, van Mierlo GJ, Muus P, Zeerleder S. Neutrophil activation and nucleosomes as markers of systemic inflammation in paroxysmal nocturnal hemoglobinuria: Effects of eculizumab. Journal of Thrombosis and Haemostasis. 2015 Nov;**13**(11):2004–2011

[96] Gupta S, Kaplan MJ. The role of neutrophils and NETosis in autoimmune and renal diseases. Nature Reviews Nephrology. 2016 Jul;**12**(7):402–413

[97] Bicker KL, Thompson PR. The protein arginine deiminases: Structure, function, inhibition, and disease. Biopolymers. 2013 Feb;**99**(2):155–163

[98] Lögters T, Margraf S, Altrichter J, Cinatl J, Mitzner S, Windolf J, Scholz M. The clinical value of neutrophil extracellular traps. Medical Microbiology and Immunology. 2009 Nov;**198**(4):211–219

[99] Papayannopoulos V, Metzler KD, Hakkim A, Zychlinsky A. Neutrophil elastase and myeloperoxidase regulate the formation of neutrophil extracellular traps. The Journal of Cell Biology. 2010 Nov;**191**(3):677–691

[100] Parker H, Dragunow M, Hampton MB, Kettle AJ, Winterbourn CC. Requirements for NADPH oxidase and myeloperoxidase in neutrophil extracellular trap formation differ depending on the stimulus. Journal of Leukocyte Biology. 2012 Oct;**92**(4):841–849

[101] Rochael NC, Guimarães-Costa AB, Nascimento MT, DeSouza-Vieira TS, Oliveira MP, Garcia e Souza LF, Oliveira MF, Saraiva EM. Classical ROS-dependent and early/rapid ROS-independent release of neutrophil extracellular traps triggered by Leishmania parasites. Scientific Reports. 2015 Dec;**5**:18302

[102] Martinod K, Witsch T, Farley K, Gallant M, Remold-O'Donnell E, Wagner DD. Neutrophil elastase-deficient mice form neutrophil extracellular traps in an experimental model of deep vein thrombosis. Journal of Thrombosis and Haemostasis. 2016 Mar;**14**(3):551–558

[103] Fuchs HJ, Borowitz DS, Christiansen DH, Morris EM, Nash ML, Ramsey BW, Rosenstein BJ, Smith AL, Wohl ME. Effect of aerosolized recombinant human DNase on exacerbations of respiratory symptoms and on pulmonary function in patients with cystic fibrosis. The Pulmozyme Study Group. The New England Journal of Medicine. 1994 Sep;**331**(10):637–642

[104] Marcos V, Zhou Z, Yildirim AO, Bohla A, Hector A, Vitkov L, Wiedenbauer EM, Krautgartner WD, Stoiber W, Belohradsky BH, Rieber N, Kormann M, Koller B, Roscher A, Roos D, Griese M, Eickelberg O, Döring G, Mall MA, Hartl D. CXCR2 mediates NADPH oxidase-independent neutrophil extracellular trap formation in cystic fibrosis airway inflammation. Nature Medicine. 2010 Sep;**16**(9):1018–1023

[105] Manzenreiter R, Kienberger F, Marcos V, Schilcher K, Krautgartner WD, Obermayer A, Huml M, Stoiber W, Hector A, Griese M, Hannig M, Studnicka M, Vitkov L, Hartl D. Ultrastructural characterization of cystic fibrosis sputum using atomic force and scanning electron microscopy. Journal of Cystic Fibrosis. 2012 Mar;**11**(2):84–92

[106] Dwyer M, Shan Q, D'Ortona S, Maurer R, Mitchell R, Olesen H, Thiel S, Huebner J, Gadjeva M. Cystic fibrosis sputum DNA has NETosis characteristics and neutrophil extracellular trap release is regulated by macrophage migration-inhibitory factor. Journal of Innate Immunity. 2014;**6**(6):765–779

[107] Yoo DG, Floyd M, Winn M, Moskowitz SM, Rada B. NET formation induced by Pseudomonas aeruginosa cystic fibrosis isolates measured as release of myeloperoxidase-DNA and neutrophil elastase-DNA complexes. Immunology Letters. 2014 Aug;**160**(2):186–194. DOI: 10.1016/j.imlet.2014.03.003. Epub23Mar2014

[108] Dubois AV, Gauthier A, Bréa D, Varaigne F, Diot P, Gauthier F, Attucci S. Influence of DNA on the activities and inhibition of neutrophil serine proteases in cystic fibrosis sputum. American Journal of Respiratory Cell and Molecular Biology. 2012 Jul;**47**(1):80–86

[109] Porto BN, Stein RT. Neutrophil extracellular traps in pulmonary diseases: Too much of a good thing? Frontiers in Immunology. 2016 Aug;**7**:311

[110] Beiter K, Wartha F, Albiger B, Normark S, Zychlinsky A, Henriques-Normark B. An endonuclease allows *Streptococcus pneumoniae* to escape from neutrophil extracellular traps. Current Biology. 2006 Feb;**16**(4):401–407

[111] Meng W, Paunel-Görgülü A, Flohé S, Hoffmann A, Witte I, MacKenzie C, Baldus SE, Windolf J, Lögters TT. Depletion of neutrophil extracellular traps in vivo results in hypersusceptibility to polymicrobial sepsis in mice. Critical Care. 2012 Jul;**16**(4):R137

[112] Jin H, Liu Z, Xiao Y, Fan X, Yan J, Liang H. Prediction of sepsis in trauma patients. Burns & Trauma. 2014 Jul;**2**(3):106–113

[113] Mohanty T, Sjögren J, Kahn F, Abu-Humaidan AH, Fisker N, Assing K, Mörgelin M, Bengtsson AA, Borregaard N, Sørensen OE. A novel mechanism for NETosis provides antimicrobial defense at the oral mucosa. Blood. 2015 Oct;**126**(18):2128–2137

[114] Sonawane S, Khanolkar V, Namavari A, Chaudhary S, Gandhi S, Tibrewal S, Jassim SH, Shaheen B, Hallak J, Horner JH, Newcomb M, Sarkar J, Jain S. Ocular surface extracellular DNA and nuclease activity imbalance: A new paradigm for inflammation in dry eye disease. Investigative Ophthalmology & Visual Science. 2012 Dec;**53**(13):8253–8263

[115] Arafat SN, Robert MC, Abud T, Spurr-Michaud S, Amparo F, Dohlman CH, Dana R, Gipson IK. Elevated neutrophil elastasein tears of ocular graft-versus-host disease patients. American Journal of Ophthalmology. 2017 Jan. pii: S0002–S9394(17)30002–8

Section 2

Neutrophil Role in Disease Pathogenesis

Chapter 4

Neutrophil Role in Periodontal Disease

Carlos Rosales and Eileen Uribe-Querol

Additional information is available at the end of the chapter

http://dx.doi.org/10.5772/67789

Abstract

Oral tissues are constantly exposed to damage from the mechanical effort of eating and from the invasion of foreign microorganisms such as bacteria, fungi, and virus. In healthy oral tissues, there is a balance between symbiotic bacteria and cells from the innate immune system, mainly neutrophils. When this balance is broken, inflammation appears and more immune cells are recruited to the gingiva. Neutrophils form a barrier against dysbiotic bacteria. However, when neutrophils are insufficient, bacteria thrive causing periodontitis, a chronic inflammatory disease that destroys the tooth-supporting tissues or periodontium. Damage of periodontal tissues leads to tooth loss, and in severe cases, it can also affect systemic health by increasing a person's risk for atherosclerosis, rheumatoid arthritis, diabetes, and even cancer. The mechanisms neutrophil employ to keep a balance with bacteria in order to maintain healthy oral tissues is the focus of this chapter. We discuss how neutrophil antimicrobial functions keep bacteria at check and how some dysbiotic bacteria block neutrophils to promote an inflammatory state. Also, novel therapeutic approaches for periodontitis are discussed.

Keywords: neutrophil, phagocytosis, degranulation, NETs, oral microbiota, dysbiotic microbiota

1. Introduction

Periodontal disease is a major public health problem due to its high prevalence worldwide [1]. Periodontitis is a more advanced inflammatory form of periodontal disease. It is a chronic inflammatory disease that causes tooth loss, by destroying the periodontium. Periodontal destruction may be caused by different factors, including accumulation of dental biofilm, poor oral hygiene, and loss of balance between oral microbiota and immune response. Dysbiosis (an alteration of oral microbiota) is thought to be the initial trigger for periodontitis [2]. The accumulation of bacteria biofilm leads to an increase in the inflammatory infiltrate, composed mainly by neutrophils into oral tissues. In this chapter, we will discuss the role of neutrophils in periodontal disease.

2. Neutrophil homeostasis

Neutrophils are considered to be the first line of defense during infections and inflammation [3]. They are the most abundant leukocytes in blood and can live for much longer than previously thought. It is estimated that neutrophils half-life is days instead of hours [4]. When microorganisms invade the organism, an inflammatory response is induced. Neutrophils are recruited from the circulation into the tissues where they destroy microorganisms by phagocytosis, by releasing antimicrobial substances, or by NETosis (**Figure 1**). This last mechanism was

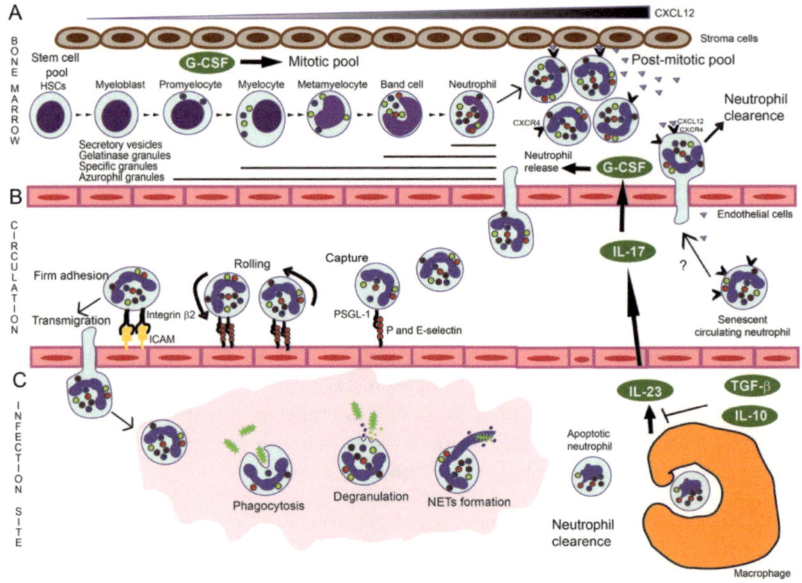

Figure 1. Neutrophil homeostasis involves production, trafficking, and clearance of these cells. (A) Production of neutrophils takes place at the bone marrow. Neutrophils maturate in the bone marrow accumulating different granules (arrow heads), azurophil, specific, and gelatinase. Finally, they also produce secretory vesicles. Lines show the moment of appearances of granules and vesicles. Neutrophils are released from the bone marrow to the circulation by interfering with the CXCR4-CXCL12 interaction. (B) Neutrophils mobilization to infection site through a leukocyte adhesion cascade that includes capture, rolling, firm adhesion, and transmigration of neutrophils (thin arrows). Senescent circulating neutrophils increase the expression of CXCR4, and respond to CXCL12 by homing back to the bone marrow. (C) Neutrophils kill bacteria by phagocytosis, degranulation, and NETs formation. Apoptotic neutrophils are cleared by macrophage phagocytosis. The process of "neutrostat" that maintains steady-state neutrophil levels (molecules with green background and green arrows). In an infected site, macrophages produce IL-23, which activates IL-17. IL-17 induces G-CSF that promotes neutrophil differentiation and release from the bone marrow (thick arrows). After macrophages phagocyte apoptotic neutrophils, they downregulate the production of IL-23 and produce IL-10 and TGF-β, this events stop the recruitment of neutrophils. CXC, chemokine receptor; IL, interleukin; G-CSF, granulocyte colony-stimulating factor.

http://dx.doi.org/10.5772/67789

recently discovered and consists on the formation of neutrophil extracellular traps (NETs) [5]. Activated neutrophils produce a variety of chemokines and cytokines, directing the inflammatory and the immune responses [6]. Unfortunately, if there is not a proper clearance of neutrophils after an infection, the proteases released from neutrophils into the surrounding tissue can cause damage to the host [7]. Bacteria biofilm deposited on teeth induces a constant recruitment of neutrophils (>95%) to the gingival sulcus (**Figure 2**) [8, 9]. Therefore, neutrophil homeostasis is important to prevent collateral damage to the host by the potent proinflammatory and antimicrobial effects of these cells. As neutrophils are the most abundant leukocytes, their excess or absence in the mouth leads to periodontal tissue damage. Moreover, neutrophil distribution and numbers are essential in maintaining oral health. Neutrophil homeostasis involves production, trafficking, and clearance of these cells [10].

2.1. Production

Thousands of neutrophils are daily produced in the bone marrow and released into the circulation [11]. Three pools of neutrophil population reside in the bone marrow: the stem cell pool, the mitotic pool, and the postmitotic pool (**Figure 1A**). The first pool consists of undifferentiated pluripotent hematopoietic stem cells (HSCs), the second pool consists of committed granulocytic progenitor cells that proliferate and differentiate. Finally, the third pool consists of fully differentiated neutrophils, which form the bone marrow reserve, available for release [12]. HSCs differentiate into myeloblasts, a developmental cell type committed to becoming granulocytes (**Figure 1A**). Granulocyte colony-stimulating factor (G-CSF) regulates both, production or granulopoiesis, and neutrophil release from the bone marrow. G-CSF regulates granulopoiesis by inducing proliferation of granulocytic precursors in the bone marrow [10]. A large postmitotic pool is retained in the bone marrow by the interaction of CXC chemokine receptor 4 (CXCR4) on neutrophils with chemokine CXCL12 (stromal-derived factor-1/SDF-1)

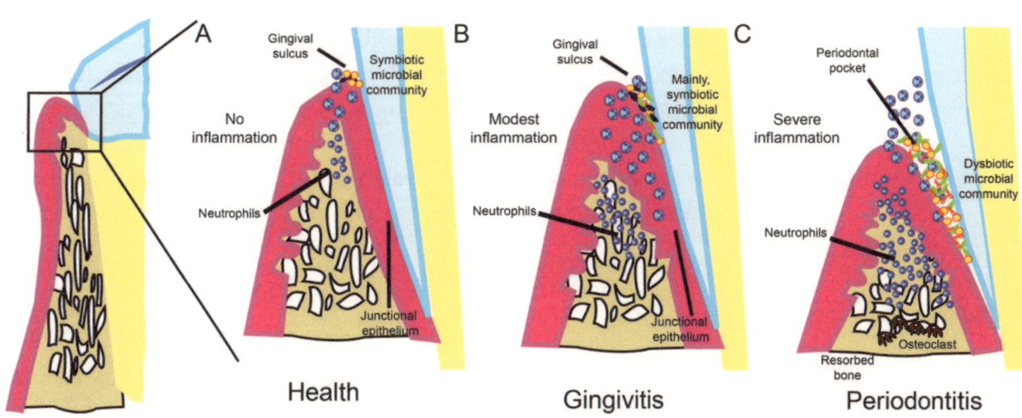

Figure 2. Neutrophil infiltrate and inflammation state. (A) In health conditions few neutrophils are recruited to the gingival sulcus to maintain symbiotic microbial community and the gum is not inflamed. (B) During gingivitis more neutrophils are recruited to the gingival sulcus and the gum in moderate inflamed. The junctional epithelium is starting to detach from the tooth. (C) During periodontitis a mayor neutrophil infiltrate is recruited to the periodontal pocket and the gum in severely inflamed. Inflammatory response activates osteoclasts, which in turn reabsorb bone.

produced by bone marrow stromal cells (**Figure 1A**). G-CSF regulates mature neutrophil release from the bone marrow by interfering with the CXCR4-CXCL12 interaction [12]. In addition, interleukin-17 (IL-17) endorses granulopoiesis and neutrophil release by upregulation of G-CSF (**Figure 1**) [10]. IL-17 builds on an interesting positive loop of neutrophil recruitment. For example, in chronic inflammation sites, neutrophils produce IL-17 and can also attract IL-17-producing $CD4^+$ T lymphocytes (Th17 cells) [13]. Neutrophils also release CCL20 and CCL2 chemokines, which are ligands for CCR6 and CCR2 chemokine receptors, respectively, on Th17 cells. This interaction maintains Th17 cells at inflammation sites. Therefore, Th17 cells secrete more IL-17 and more neutrophils are recruited [14].

2.2. Trafficking

Circulating neutrophils can be quickly mobilized to infection or inflammation sites through a systematically controlled process known as the leukocyte adhesion cascade, which achieves neutrophil transmigration (**Figure 1B**) [15]. The process initiates when endothelial cells get activated and upregulated the expression of adhesion receptors such as E- and P-selectins. Neutrophils recognize these selectins and begin rolling on endothelial cells. This rolling depends on transient interactions of selectins with glycoprotein ligands on neutrophils. Next, neutrophils get activated by chemokines, which induce a high affinity state in integrins, another group of adhesion receptors. Interaction of both selectins and integrins with their corresponding ligands leads to slow neutrophils rolling followed by a firm adhesion that brings neutrophils to a full stop. Finally, neutrophils crawl on the endothelium and transmigrate into infection or inflammation sites. This last process is regulated mainly by $\beta 2$ integrins. Integrins are heterodimeric receptors formed by a unique α (CD11) and a common β (CD18) subunit that interact with adhesion ligands such as intercellular adhesion molecule-1 (ICAM-1) and ICAM-2 on endothelial cells (**Figure 1B**). This leukocyte adhesion cascade is positive regulated by tissue-derived cytokines and by tissue-derived chemokines. Cytokines control the expression of endothelial adhesion molecules and chemokines induce integrins to change conformation into a high affinity state [16]. Once neutrophils move into tissues, they follow chemoattractant gradients to reach infection or inflammation sites. Some chemoattractants for neutrophils are activated by complement components, such as the anaphylatoxin C5a, and bacterial components, such as formyl-methionyl-leucyl-phenylalanine (fMLF). Recently, it has been discovered that the leukocyte adhesion cascade is also negatively regulated by endogenous inhibitors such as Del-1 (developmental endothelial locus-1), pentraxin 3, and growth-differentiation factor 15 [17].

2.3. Clearance

Neutrophils are mostly cleared in tissues (**Figure 1C**) and possibly also in the bone marrow (**Figure 1A**). In tissues, once neutrophils have completed their antimicrobial duty, they undergo apoptosis. Resident phagocytes, for instance, macrophages and dendritic cells, clear neutrophils locally. Phagocytosis of apoptotic neutrophils reprograms macrophages to initiate an anti-inflammatory response, characterized by the synthesis of tumor growth factor (TGF)-β and IL-10, and by a reduction in IL-23 synthesis (**Figure 1**) [18]. IL-23 cytokine induces IL-17 synthesis; thus, the reduced IL-17 levels lead to less

G-CSF production and in consequence, less neutrophil production. This process is a control loop that has been described as a "neutrostat" (neutrophil rheostat), and maintains steady-state neutrophil levels (**Figure 1**) [14]. Senescent circulating neutrophils are recruited for clearance in the bone marrow. These neutrophils increase the expression of CXCR4, and respond to CXCL12 by homing back to the bone marrow (**Figure 1**) [19]. Apoptosis and proper removal of apoptotic cells are key aspects of inflammation resolution. Neutrophils death is influenced by environmental conditions including hypoxia and presence of inflammatory mediators, such as granulocyte/monocyte colony-stimulating factor (GM-CSF) and lipopolysaccharides (LPS). Neutrophil clearance depends on signals that apoptotic neutrophils express on their surface. These signals allow macrophages to recognize and ingest the neutrophils (**Figure 1C**) [20]. Failure to clear these apoptotic cells results in secondary necrosis and release of products that generate proinflammatory signals. Neutrophils express molecules that regulate their survival. Some of these molecules are survivin, cyclin-dependent kinases and proliferating cell nuclear antigen (PCNA). Survivin is expressed more highly in immature neutrophils than in mature ones, but its expression can be reestablished in mature cells by inflammatory signals, for instance, GM-CSF or G-CSF [21]. Similarly, cyclin-dependent kinases function as prosurvival factors. Their inhibition induces caspase-dependent apoptosis. PCNA in neutrophils associates with procaspases in the cytosol and is thought to prevent their activation. During apoptosis, PCNA is targeted for proteosomal degradation, which correlates with an increase in caspase-3 and caspase-8 activities [11].

3. Neutrophils in oral health

Commonly, it is thought that microbes are harmful to our health. Contrary to this thought, there are plenty of microbes that harmoniously live within our bodies and form our microbiota. Homeostasis between the host and its symbiotic microbiota is a key factor to understand and maintain our health [22, 23]. Nevertheless, we are constantly exposed to microbes not belonging to our microbiota through the things we touch, the food we eat, and the air we inhale. Fortunately, our innate immune system protects us from this constant threat. The oral cavity is a special place, where the microbiota is constantly changing. Yet, homeostatic mechanisms exist that keep the oral microbiota in balance with the immune system. Neutrophils are actively recruited into the gingival sulcus by an interleukin (IL)-8 gradient continuously secreted by the junctional epithelium, as this tissue is in close contact with the oral biofilm bacterial community (**Figure 2**). Neutrophils are mostly responsible for ensuring periodontal health by keeping this biofilm at check [24]. However, during gingivitis a moderate inflammatory response is generated. If this inflammation is not controlled, for example, in situations or poor oral hygiene, gingivitis can lead to periodontitis, a chronic inflammatory disease. In this condition, microbial pathogens cannot be eliminated or controlled by neutrophils. In response, more neutrophils are recruited to the periodontal tissue. Neutrophil accumulation, instead of protecting, favors periodontal tissue damage and even bone loss (**Figure 2**). Thus, a close balance between neutrophil function and microbe challenge must be maintained to ensure periodontal health.

4. Antimicrobial mechanisms of neutrophils

Neutrophils are equipped with different antimicrobial mechanisms, which help them to fight a broad spectrum of bacteria, fungi, and protozoa. These mechanisms include phagocytosis, degranulation, and neutrophil extracellular traps (NETs) (**Figure 1**).

4.1. Phagocytosis

Phagocytosis is a receptor-mediated process during which a particle is internalized by the cell into a vacuole called the phagosome. Neutrophils recognize pathogens through pattern-recognition receptors (PAMPs), or opsonins (antibody molecules or complement components). Opsonized pathogens are efficiently phagocytosed when they bind with antibody receptors (Fc receptors) or complement receptors on the neutrophil (**Figure 3**). After engulfment, the nascent phagosome matures by fusing with lysosomes. This brings antimicrobial molecules into the phagosomal lumen. The vesicle is now called phagolysosome. Concurrently, reactive oxygen species (ROS) production starts by the assembly of the NADPH oxidase on the phagosomal membrane, and the pH inside the phagosome drops to 4.5–5. Also, potassium ions (K^+) are pumped into the phagolysosome; this K^+ influx mediates the release of serine proteases. In addition, hydrogen peroxide (H_2O_2) is also converted into hypochloric acid (HOCl) in a reaction catalyzed by myeloperoxidase (MPO) [25]. Granules content and ROS create an environment toxic to the pathogen. Unfortunately, not all pathogens are killed inside the phagosome. Moreover, some have advanced strategies to survive inside neutrophils. These strategies include interfering with engulfment, modulating phagosome maturation, and creating a more hospitable intraphagosomal environment.

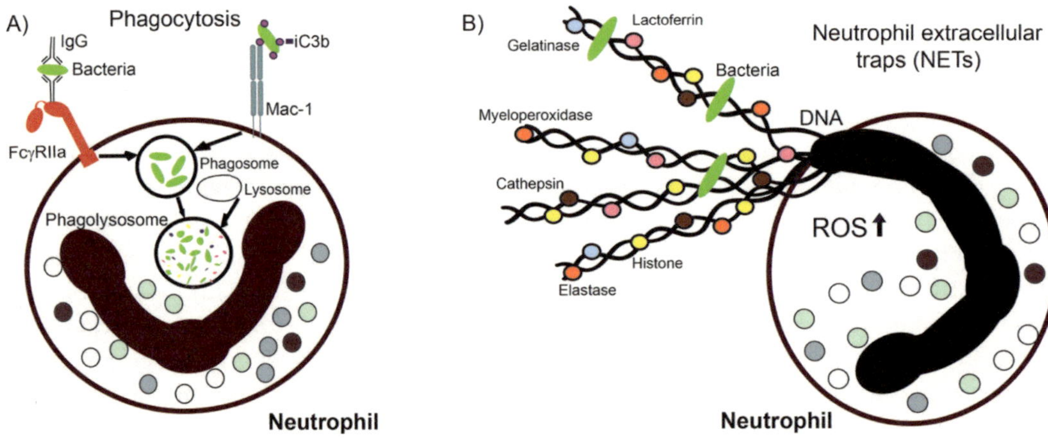

Figure 3. Phagocytosis and NETs. (A) Neutrophils recognize opsonized pathogens through Fc Receptors (FcγRIIa) or complement receptors (Mac-1) on their membrane. The pathogen is internalized into a nascent phagosome, which matures by fusing with lysosomes forming a phagolysosome. (B) Neutrophil extracellular traps (NETs) are formed when neutrophils release decondensed chromatin decorated with antimicrobial molecules, into the extracellular space. ROS, reactive oxygen species.

4.2. Degranulation

In the bone marrow, as precursor cells mature into neutrophils, they synthesize proteins that are sorted into different granules [26]. Granules formation begins in early promyelocytes and continues throughout the various stages of myeloid cell development. The granules are arbitrarily subdivided into three different classes based on their resident cargo molecules: azurophilic, specific, and gelatinase granules (**Figure 1A**, **Table 1**). Neutrophils also form secretory vesicles until the last step of their differentiation (**Figure 1A**, **Table 1**). Granule heterogeneity is explained by regulated expression of the granule protein genes. This regulation is mediated by the combination of myeloid transcription factors that express at specific stages of neutrophil development. Vesicle availability and exocytosis depends on mobilizable intracellular compartments of the neutrophil. Mature neutrophils are released into the circulation and, in response to infection, they leave the circulation and migrate toward the inflammatory site. Exocytosis of granules and secretory vesicles plays a crucial role in most neutrophil functions from early activation to the destruction of phagocytosed microorganisms. Secretory vesicles have the highest propensity for extracellular release, followed by gelatinase granules, specific granules, and azurophil granules [27, 28]. For example, neutrophil stimulation with phorbol myristate acetate (PMA) induces complete release of gelatinase granules, restrained release of specific granules, and minimal exocytosis of azurophil granules. In a different way, neutrophil stimulation with fMLF induces release of mostly secretory vesicles without

Azurophil granules	Specific granules	Gelatinase granules	Secretory vesicles
Azurocidin	CD11b/CD18	Acetyltransferase	Alkaline phosphatase
Bacterial/permeability-increasing protein	Cathelicidin	CD11b/CD18	CD11b/CD18 (CR3)
	Collagenase	Cytochrome b558	CD14
Cathepsins	Cytochrome b558	Gelatinase	CD16
Defensins	fMLP-R	Leukolysin	CR1
Lysozyme	Lactoferrin	Lysozyme	Cytochrome b558
Myeloperoxidase	Leukolysin	Natural-resistance-associated macrophage protein 1 (NRAMP1)	FRP
Natural serine proteases	Lysozyme		fMLF-R
Cathepsin G	Neutrophil gelatinase-associated lipocalin (NGAL)		
Neutrophil elastase			
Proteinase 3			

Note: CR, complement receptor; FPR, formyl peptide receptor; NGAL, neutrophil gelatinase-associated lipocalin; NRAMP1, natural-resistance-associated macrophage protein 1.

Table 1. Cytoplasmic granules of neutrophils [24–26, 28].

significant release of granules. The hierarchical mobilization of neutrophil granules and secretory vesicles depends on intracellular Ca^{2+} level. Gradual elevations in intracellular Ca^{2+} are induced by ligation of L-selectin, CD11b/CD18, and the fMLP receptors [26].

4.3. Neutrophil extracellular traps (NETs)

Neutrophil stimulation can also undergo a mechanism called NETosis. Although NETosis has previously been described as a special form of programmed cell death, there are forms of NET production that do not end with the demise of neutrophils. NETosis leads to the release of decondensed chromatin into the extracellular space. The chromatin forms a trap for pathogens that looks like a net, which is why they are called neutrophil extracellular traps (NETs). NETs also contain histones, cytoplasmic proteins, and antimicrobial granular molecules. NETs formation mechanisms are still unknown, nevertheless, NADPH oxidase activation, reactive oxygen species (ROS) production, myeloperoxidase (MPO), and neutrophil elastase (NE) release (**Figure 3**) are required [25].

5. Neutrophil interactions with symbiotic oral bacteria

In periodontal health, the interaction between symbiotic microbial community and neutrophils is strongly controlled to prevent tissue damage. This interaction has been evaluated in studies with germ-free mice and specific pathogen-free mice. Results of these studies showed that oral symbiotic commensal microbiota has no impact on the structure of gingival tissue of germ-free mice, while gut commensal microbiota is fundamental on the structural formation of the intestinal tissue [29]. Periodontal tissue recruits neutrophils by means of the chemotactic receptor CXCR2. This receptor has two ligands CXCL1 and CXCL2. Both ligands are expressed in the junctional epithelium of germ-free and specific pathogen-free mice, but there is a significant increase on CXCL2 in the epithelium of specific pathogen-free mice. Therefore, oral bacterial community induces an increase in neutrophil recruitment via CXCL2 [29]. Neutrophils play a key role in preserving oral health, since low neutrophil counts as well as deficiency in neutrophil functional responses have been associated with periodontal disease. As mentioned before, neutrophils kill pathogens by phagocytosis, degranulation, or NETs formation (**Figure 1C**). Neutrophils are very efficient phagocytic cells and have a very efficient antimicrobial mechanism to do so, the respiratory burst response. In this response, high consumption of oxygen results in the production of reactive oxygen species (ROS), through the activation of the NADPH oxidase complex (**Figure 3**) [5]. Patients with chronic granulomatous disease, a rare genetic disorder that consist on mutations in the NADPH oxidase, are inefficient in mounting a respiratory burst response. As a consequence, these patients present early in life recurrent infections [30]. These patients present higher bacteria colonization and gingivitis; however, they do not present periodontitis [31].

6. The evolution from a healthy periodontium to periodontitis

In the oral cavity, the tooth surface offers a niche for bacteria colonization and biofilm formation resulting in a varied polymicrobial community. A healthy environment is maintained if the

http://dx.doi.org/10.5772/67789

multiplication of symbiotic microbiota is regulated. Periodontal diseases are related to a shift from symbiotic microbiota to dysbiotic microbiota, and this shift is related with the accumulation of dental plaque or biofilm. Biofilm elaboration consists of four sequential phases. Phase 1 consists of the adsorption of different molecules to a surface to condition the biofilm formation. Phase 2 consists of single organism adhesion. Phase 3 consists of growth of extracellular matrix production and multiplication of adhering bacteria and phase 4 consists of sequential adsorption of further bacteria to form a more complex and mature biofilm (**Figure 4**) [32]. The microbial etiology of gingivitis and periodontitis has been established for several decades. In 1994, Haffajee and Socransky adapted Koch's postulates to be used in the identification of periodontal pathogens. In 1996, at the World Workshop in Periodontics three species of pathogens were identified as causative factors of periodontitis *Aggregatibacter actinomycetemcomitans*, *Porphyromonas gingivalis*, and *Tannerella forsythia*; however, these three species cannot be considered to be the only causative pathogens of periodontitis, but we are certain that they participate in the disease [32].

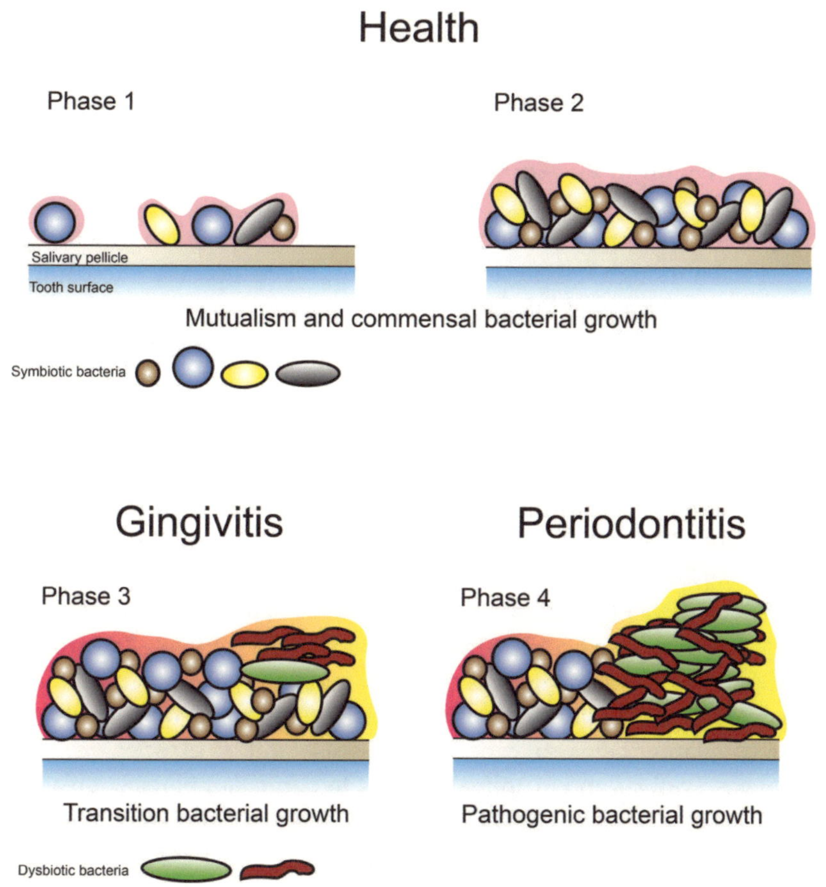

Figure 4. Biofilm elaboration consists of four sequential phases. Phase 1 consists of the adsorption of different molecules to a surface to condition the biofilm formation. Phase 2 consists of single organism adhesion. Phase 3 consists of growth of extracellular matrix production and multiplication of adhering bacteria and phase 4 consists of sequential adsorption of further bacteria to form a more complex and mature biofilm. The first two phases are representative of health, phase 3 of gingivitis, and phase 4 of periodontitis.

6.1. Balanced inflammation

Neutrophils are the main leukocytes recruited to the gingival sulcus. Neutrophils exit the gingival blood vessels and travel through the gingival junctional epithelium until they reach the sulcus [8]. In the sulcus, neutrophils create a barrier against the growing bacteria biofilm to prevent bacteria from invading the underlying tissues. Neutrophil migration from vessels toward the gingival sulcus requires CXCR2 binding to CXCL2. Migration is controlled by gradients of chemokines and adhesion molecules such as IL-8, ICAM-1, and E-selectin [29]. Neutrophil presence in the sulcus is necessary to preserve oral health since patients with altered neutrophil production and distribution develop severe periodontitis at early ages [33]. Chédiak-Higashi syndrome, Papillon-Lefèvre syndrome, neutropenias, and leukocyte adhesion deficiency (LAD) are some examples of neutrophil diseases. In Papillon-Lefèvre syndrome neutrophils have defective chemotaxis, as a consequence, they are not efficiently recruited to the sites of inflammation and infection [34]. Neutropenia, a persistent reduction of neutrophil numbers in circulation, is frequently associated with susceptibility to infections. In many neutropenic conditions, severe periodontal disease is recurrently seen since primary dentition eruption [35]. CXCR2-deficient mice cannot recruit neutrophils to oral tissues. These mice also experience periodontitis and periodontal bone loss early in life [36]. Leukocyte adhesion deficiency is a group of inherited disorders, in which neutrophils fail to transmigrate from the circulation to the site of inflammation or infection. Neutrophils of patients with leukocyte adhesion deficiency have defective expression and function of adhesion molecules like integrins. Therefore, neutrophils cannot adhere firmly to the vascular endothelium to transmigrate. Even though the presence of neutrophils is necessary to control infections, plenty of neutrophils on a site of infection is not always protective. In fact, neutrophil numbers in inflamed periodontal tissues correlate with the severity of the lesions [37], and tissue destruction seems to be a collateral damage of hyperactive neutrophils [38].

6.2. Periodontitis

Periodontal diseases cause the destruction of the tooth supporting tissues, gingiva, periodontal ligament, cement, and alveolar bone and may eventually lead to tooth loss. Severe periodontitis affects approximately 10% of the global population [39]. Periodontal disease is the consequence of a shift in oral microbiota population from a symbiotic to a dysbiotic microbial community in the mouth. Periodontal disease begins when some factors that promote the growth of selected symbiotic bacteria, induce host inflammatory pathways [40, 41]. Periodontitis not only severely deteriorates people's quality of life by impairing the dentition but also adversely affect systemic health. A clear correlation between periodontal disease and atherosclerosis has been established in clinical observations and in animal models. In particular, polymicrobial infection with *Treponema denticola, Porphyromonas gingivalis, Tannerella forsythia,* and *Fusobacterium nucleatum* has been shown to promote progression of atherosclerosis [42]. Another correlation between periodontitis and diabetes also has been well documented. Higher plaque levels and higher incidence of chronic gingivitis are both found in adults and in children with diabetes [43, 44]. Periodontal treatment showed a beneficial effect on metabolic control of type 2 diabetic patients. Other various systemic diseases such as diabetes, cardiac disease, low birth weight, renal diseases, metabolic syndrome, obesity, Parkinson's disease, and Alzheimer's disease have been also proposed to be linked with periodontal disease on the basis of systemic inflammation [40, 41, 45].

6.3. Inflammation in periodontitis

Periodontitis is associated with a change in oral microbiota from symbiotic bacteria to dysbiotic anaerobic microorganisms, which have adapted to succeed in an inflammatory environment (**Figure 4**). Pathogenic bacteria, such as *Porphyromonas gingivalis*, induce changes in the normal microbiota of the gingival crevicular fluid, leading to increased biofilm deposition in the gingival sulcus. The gingival sulcus is the space between the tooth surface and the free gingiva. Pathogenic bacteria also induce moderate inflammation known as gingivitis (**Figure 4**). When this moderate inflammation is not well resolved, a chronic inflammatory state is established, which results in the formation of pathologically deepened gingival sulcus also called periodontal pockets, followed by extensive tissue destruction, including bone loss (**Figures 2** and **4**). These last events are induced by the accumulation of dysbiotic bacteria in the periodontal pockets and are thought to be the initial trigger for periodontitis [46]. Accumulation of dysbiotic bacteria biofilm leads to an increase in the inflammatory infiltrate, composed mainly by neutrophils into oral tissues. There, neutrophils form a barrier that prevents bacteria from invading deeper tissues and are essential for maintaining healthy oral tissues. In the case of neutrophils deficiencies, severe periodontitis appears with a concomitant inflammation state. On the contrary, excess numbers of neutrophils induces a chronic inflammatory state. Thus, inflammation is an important element in periodontitis that is deregulated when neutrophil homeostasis is altered. Periodontitis in the absence of neutrophils has traditionally been explained by the lack of neutrophil control on bacterial infections. Patients with leukocyte adhesion deficiency present frequent infections and develop early severe periodontitis. However, this type of periodontitis does not usually respond to treatment with antibiotics or mechanical removal of bacteria biofilm, suggesting that other mechanisms are at work. Recently it was shown that the driving force for this type of periodontitis involves the production of IL-23 and IL-17. In leukocyte adhesion deficiency type 1 patients, T cells were identified as the main producers of IL-17 [47]. IL-17 not only stimulates fibroblasts to produce G-CSF but also promotes inflammation and stimulates osteoclasts, leading to bone loss. These findings are in agreement with the neutrostat mechanism discussed above. When apoptotic neutrophils are phagocytosed by macrophages, anti-inflammatory signals are produced that lead to less IL-23 production, which is a strong inducer for IL-17 production. IL-17 in turn induces G-CSF production (**Figure 1**).

Neutrophils can be found in large numbers in inflamed periodontal tissues, and their presence correlates with the severity of the periodontal destruction. Therefore, this destruction seems to be collateral damage of hyperactive neutrophils [48, 49]. Neutrophil recruitment is at least in part regulated by Del-1 and LFA-1 interactions. Del-1 blocks LFA-1 binding to its ligand ICAM-1 and prevents neutrophil transmigration [50]. Neutrophil recruitment is also triggered with elevated IL-17 levels, which resulted to be responsible for the tissue damage, because antibodies against IL-17 prevented inflammation and bone loss. High levels of IL-17 could be responsible for the bone loss in chronic periodontitis, by stimulating osteoblast expression of RANKL, an important osteoclastogenesis factor.

6.4. Dysbiotic bacteria

Diverse environments present in the oral cavity allow symbiotic and dysbiotic microbiota to find the best niche that fits their growth requirements, resulting in the formation of unique microbial biofilm communities. Periodontal disease microbiota includes a large number of microorganisms including *P. gingivalis, Tannerella forsythia,* and *Treponema denticola* [51]. Fortunately, nucleic acid screening and 16S pyrosequencing techniques have made more efficient finding changes in microbiota of healthy and of periodontal disease patients [52]. Screenings have been made at nine different oral sites including the oral epithelium, the maxillary anterior vestibule, the dorsum and lateral tongue surface, the hard and soft palate, the tonsils, the tooth surfaces, and the subgingival plaque [53, 54]. There are between 100 and 300 bacterial species in a single individual. Our general idea is that infectious diseases are caused by the action of a single foreign pathogen. However, periodontitis is originated by the complex association and interaction of a diverse polymicrobial community [37, 51, 55]. Data obtained from oral biofilm studies using checkerboard DNA-DNA techniques link the different stages of the disease to a specific bacterial group or complex with the presence of the triad of bacteria composed by *P. gingivalis, T. forsythia,* and *T. denticola,* which are strongly associated with increased severity of periodontitis [56]. Other microorganisms have also been identified such as *F. alocis,* a Gram-positive bacterium, which is present in periodontal disease sites, while *Veillonella sp,* a Gram-negative uncultivated bacterium, is associated with healthy periodontal sites. This data indicates that the general idea of Gram-negative anaerobic bacteria being the pathogen population is not completely correct.

In a healthy gingival tissue, the local symbiotic microbiota is less diverse and rich, with neutrophil recruitment to clear the infection and resolving the inflammation with no collateral damage to the host (**Figures 4** and **5**). The progression from health to periodontitis is now explained as the transition from a symbiotic microbiota to a polymicrobial dysbiotic microbiota. Several risks factors, such as smoking, tissue injury, diet changes, an immunocompromised host, or the colonization of the oral cavity by pathogenic bacteria can modify the oral ecosystem resulting in a dysbiotic polymicrobial community. In consequence, the host's response toward the polymicrobial dysbiotic microbiota challenge is more robust and not regulated, transitioning from a controlled/stable immune response into a nonresolving chronic inflammatory response [57].

Polymicrobial dysbiotic microbiota has an arsenal of self-defense mechanisms, which can be directed to attack against neutrophils or camouflage the biofilm (**Figure 5**) [58]. Microbiota has an intermicrobial communication called quorum sensing, that enables the dysbiotic microbiota to optimize the biofilm conditions and ensure nutrient supply. Among the defense mechanisms, the production of bacterial surfactants by *P. aeruginosa* biofilms causes rapid cell death in neutrophils [59]. Additionally, quorum sensing molecules control neutrophil ROS response and penetration into *P. aeruginosa* biofilms [60]. Similarly, *Aggregatibacter actinomycetemcomitans* and *S. aureus* produce bacterial toxins that induce neutrophils lysis and degranulation [61–63]. In addition to directly attacking neutrophils, dysbiotic microbiota in biofilms can render themselves resistant to neutrophil-mediated killing by disguising their immunogenicity. NET formation within *Haemophilus influenzae* biofilms does not harm the biofilm. This is presumably due to their expression of certain lipooligosaccharide glycoforms, which shield pathogen-associated molecular patterns (PAMPs) and thus inhibit recognition and

http://dx.doi.org/10.5772/67789

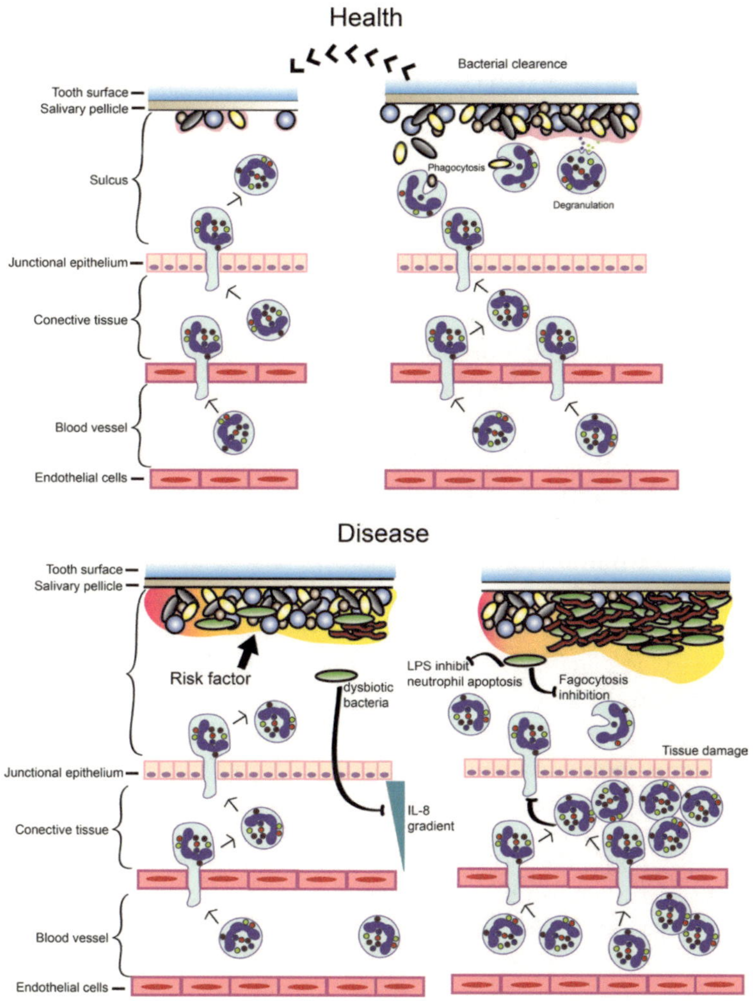

Figure 5. Neutrophil response in periodontal health and disease. Health: Symbiotic bacteria community adheres to molecules of the salivary pellicle that are bound to the tooth surface. Few neutrophils patrol the gingival sulcus, and as the bacterial burden increases, neutrophils regularly exit the blood stream entering the connective tissue layer beneath the junctional epithelium and the tooth and kill some of the associated microbes (thin arrows). Neutrophils maintain bacterial concentration so there is no inflammation or tissue damage (arrow heads). Disease: Following the presence of a risk factor (smoking, poor diet, injury, etc.; thick arrow) dysbiotic bacteria (big oval) can colonize the symbiotic microbial community. Following colonization, the sulcus is invaded by dysbiotic bacteria which shut down the IL-8 production. Neutrophils enter the connective tissue, but do not get to the sulcus. This causes many neutrophils to accumulate in the connective tissue. As some neutrophils transmigrate to the dysbiotic biofilm increase inflammation is conducted by neutrophil degranulation, reactive oxygen species (ROS) production, and NETosis that damages the host tissue.

opsonization. This molecule can provide protection against antimicrobial peptides [64]. One important microbial defense mechanism is the evasion of phagocytosis. Prevotella strains were recognized by neutrophils but not phagocytosed, depending on whether they produced mannose-rich exopolysaccharides as part of their extracellular matrix [65]. *S. aureus* is able to survive after being phagocytosed by neutrophils [66]. *S. aureus* is known to be potent triggers for NETosis and degranulation. Therefore, it can be assumed that implementation of such survival strategies coexists with the elimination of bacteria by neutrophils. Finally, inflammation and tissue destruction mediated by neutrophils evoke frequent gingival bleeding, which these bacteria may use as an additional source of nutrients, such as iron and vitamin K.

7. *Porphyromonas gingivalis*

Porphyromonas gingivalis are anaerobic, Gram-negative, nonmotile, asaccharolytic rods that usually exhibit coccal or short rod morphologies. It is part of the black-pigmented Bacteriodes group [32]. *P. gingivalis*, even in low colonization levels, can induce the shift from symbiotic microbiota to dysbiotic microbiota followed by inflammatory bone loss. This bacteria uses different mechanisms to destabilize neutrophil homeostasis, inhibition of phagocytic killing, resistance to granule-derived antimicrobial agents and to the oxidative burst, impaired recruitment and chemotaxis, promote inflammatory response, and delay of neutrophil apoptosis. *P. gingivalis* has a number of virulence factors related to the subversion of the innate immune system. This ability is what often characterizes a successful pathogen, as it tends to disable the overall host response while simultaneously enhancing the pathogenicity of a polymicrobial community. *P. gingivalis* are resistant to oxidative killing [67] and recruit hyperactive neutrophils with an enhanced response, which is characterized by the release of reactive oxygen intermediates, several cationic peptides, and enzymes such as matrix metalloproteinases (MMPs). All this responses increased tissue damage [48]. *P. gingivalis* also can manipulate both complement and TLR signaling to induce bacterial persistence.

Porphyromonas gingivalis gingipains are able to trigger the expression of proinflammatory surface receptor TREM-1 on neutrophils, and several periodontopathogenic species can induce IL-8 gene expression in gingival epithelial cells and fibroblasts [68, 69].

8. *Treponema denticola*

Treponema denticola is an anaerobic, Gram-negative, motile, spirochete that can be poorly detected in the gingival plaque of healthy individuals. However, it is present in very high numbers in the subgingival periodontal pocket and is associated with the dysbiotic microbiota biofilm formation in periodontal lesions. *T. denticola* limits neutrophil chemotaxis, and inhibits junctional epithelial cells to secrete IL-8. Additionally, this pathogen is able to degrade IL-8 that is already present at the infection site, which disables the neutrophil chemotactic gradient. *T. denticola* major outer sheath protein (Msp) is one of its most important virulence factors in contributing to the disease progression. This membrane protein modulates neutrophil signaling pathways involved in cytoskeletal dynamics that are relevant in chemotaxis and phagocytosis [70]. Msp controls neutrophil cytoskeletal functions like migration, adhesion, and cell shape. It also causes extracellular matrix degradation by stimulating the release of activated MMPs from neutrophils.

9. Neutrophil persistence and chronic inflammation

Neutrophils are recruited to infection and inflammation sites by different chemoattractants such as interleukin 8 (IL-8), complement fragment C5a, or chemokine CXCL5. They migrate through the junctional epithelium and finally arrive in the gingival sulcus and in gingival crevicular fluid. Neutrophils in saliva retain their phagocytic function, and their ability to generate ROS [71, 72]. NETs containing trapped bacteria have been described within the gingival sulcus, in purulent periodontal pockets, and on the surface of gingival epithelial cells. On condition that neutrophils and NETs do not occur excessively and are rapidly cleared, relatively little damage to the adjacent tissues is induced. Nevertheless, it has been widely reported that neutrophils can be responsible for both host defense and host tissue damage. Release of proteolytic and collagenolytic enzymes as well as ROS within host tissues, often lead to extracellular matrix degradation and persistent inflammation, are the main causes of tissue damage. Normally, connective tissue is degraded to allow fast transmigration of neutrophils and other cells involved in wound healing but during periodontitis it produces a chronic inflammatory disease. Hence, inflammation overweighs resolution, and host tissue destruction becomes progressive, eventually resulting in pathological osteolysis and tooth loss [58].

10. Therapeutic approaches

As it was discussed along this chapter, it is clear that both, lack of neutrophils and excess of neutrophils in the periodontium, can lead to periodontal disease. Because both situations involve IL-17-mediated inflammation and bone loss, it is conceivable that IL-17 or IL-17R inhibitors may be promising targets for treatment of human periodontitis. By blocking IL-17 actions, neutrophil recruitment to the periodontium would be reduced and in consequence, the inflammation state would also be reduced. This should prevent tissue damage and loss of bone.

In chronic periodontitis, periodontal bacteria activate neutrophil subversion pathways that allow bacteria to escape neutrophil killing. For example, *P. aeruginosa* biofilms produce bacterial surfactants that induce rapid neutrophil death [59], and *Aggregatibacter actinomycetemcomitans* and *S. aureus* produce bacterial toxins that induce neutrophil lysis and degranulation [61–63]. These bacterial products could be neutralized with antibodies or novel pharmaceutical drugs to prevent their negative effects on neutrophils. Also, *P. gingivalis* can manipulate complement to induce bacterial persistence. Thus, complement components are also good therapeutic targets. In fact, in preclinical models of periodontitis the use of complement inhibitors has led to a reduction of the inflammatory state [73, 74]. In addition, several bacteria including *P. gingivalis* can induce cells such as fibroblasts to produce IL-8 and recruit more neutrophils to the inflamed periodontal tissues [68, 69]. Blocking IL-8 is another interesting therapeutic strategy for reducing periodontitis. Several anti-IL-8 blocking antibodies are available. Their potential benefit in periodontal disease should be evaluated in the near future.

Del-1 is another promising candidate molecule to be used therapeutically to prevent neutrophil recruitment and bone loss associated with periodontal inflammation [17]. Since Del-1 blocks LFA-1 binding to its ligand ICAM-1 and prevents neutrophil transmigration [50], it could be administered to inflamed tissues, to reduce neutrophil recruitment, and to reduce inflammation. In fact, this is exactly what was found in a model of periodontitis with nonhuman primates [75]. Local administration of Del-1 also prevented inflammatory bone loss [75]. Preclinical studies for the use of Del-1 are now underway.

All these potential therapeutic approaches promise a relief from periodontitis and perhaps other inflammatory disorders in the future.

11. Conclusion

Neutrophils are specialized phagocytes that coordinate and execute inflammation. Neutrophils constantly surveil oral tissues in order to guarantee oral health. Alterations in the neutrophil homeostasis (defects in recruitment and proper function) lead to periodontal diseases. Also, hyperactive neutrophils can exacerbate and even cause autoimmune and inflammatory diseases. Chronic infections driven by pathogenic biofilms indicate that the immune system fails to fully protect the host. New potential therapeutic approaches have been identified. They promise a relief from periodontitis and perhaps other inflammatory disorders.

Acknowledgements

This work was supported by Grant 254434 from Consejo Nacional de Ciencia y Tecnología, México (to Carlos Rosales), and by Grant PAPIIT IA202013 (to Eileen Uribe-Querol) from Dirección General de Asuntos del Personal Académico, Universidad Nacional Autónoma de México, Mexico.

Author details

Carlos Rosales[1] and Eileen Uribe-Querol[2*]

*Address all correspondence to: euquerol@comunidad.unam.mx

1 Immunology Department, Instituto de Investigaciones Biomédicas, Universidad Nacional Autónoma de México, Mexico City, Mexico

2 Advanced Research Division, Facultad de Odontología, Universidad Nacional Autónoma de México, Mexico City, Mexico

References

[1] Petersen PE, Ogawa H: The global burden of periodontal disease: towards integration with chronic disease prevention and control. Periodontol. 2000 2012; 60:15–39. DOI: 10.1111/j.1600-0757.2011.00425.x.

[2] Rosier BT, De Jager M, Zaura E, Krom BP: Historical and contemporary hypotheses on the development of oral diseases: are we there yet? Front. Cell. Infect. Microbiol. 2014; 4:92. DOI: 10.3389/fcimb.2014.00092

[3] Borregaard N: Neutrophils, from marrow to microbes. Immunity 2010; 33:657–670. DOI: 10.1016/j.immuni.2010.11.011

[4] Tak T, Tesselaar K, Pillay J, Borghans JA, Koenderman L, Tesselaar K, Pillay J, Borghans JA, Koenderman L: What's your age again? Determination of human neutrophil half-lives revisited. J. Leukoc. Biol. 2013; 94:595–601. DOI: 10.1189/jlb.1112571

[5] Nauseef WM: How human neutrophils kill and degrade microbes: an integrated view. Immunol. Rev. 2007 219:88–102. DOI: 10.1111/j.1600-065X.2007.00550.x

[6] Mócsai A: Diverse novel functions of neutrophils in immunity, inflammation, and beyond. J. Exp. Med. 2013; 210:1283–1299. DOI: 10.1084/jem.20122220.

[7] Mayadas TN, Cullere X, Lowell CA: The multifaceted functions of neutrophils. Annu. Rev. Pathol. 2014; 9:181–218. DOI: 10.1146/annurev-pathol-020712-164023

[8] Hajishengallis E, Hajishengallis G: Neutrophil homeostasis and periodontal health in children and adults. J. Dent. Res. 2014 93:231–237. DOI: 10.1177/0022034513507956

[9] Delima AJ, Van Dyke TE: Origin and function of the cellular components in gingival crevice fluid. Periodontol. 2000. 2003; 31:55–76.

[10] von Vietinghoff S, Ley K: Homeostatic regulation of blood neutrophil counts. J. Immunol. 2008; 181:5183–5188.

[11] Amulic B, Cazalet C, Hayes GL, Metzler KD, Zychlinsky A: Neutrophil function: from mechanisms to disease. Annu. Rev. Immunol. 2012; 30:459–489. DOI: 10.1146/annurev-immunol-020711-074942

[12] Summers C, Rankin SM, Condliffe AM, Singh N, Peters AM, Chilvers ER: Neutrophil kinetics in health and disease. Trends Immunol. 2010; 31:318–324. DOI: 10.1016/j.it.2010.05.006.

[13] Weaver CT, Elson CO, Fouser LA, Kolls JK: The Th17 pathway and inflammatory diseases of the intestines, lungs, and skin. Annu. Rev. Pathol. 2013; 8:477–512. DOI: 10.1146/annurev-pathol-011110-130318

[14] Cortés-Vieyra R, Rosales C, Uribe-Querol E: Neutrophil functions in periodontal homeostasis. J. Immunol. Res. 2016; 2016:1396106. DOI: 10.1155/2016/1396106

[15] Ley K, Laudanna C, Cybulsky MI, Nourshargh S: Getting to the site of inflammation: the leukocyte adhesion cascade updated. Nat. Rev. Immunol. 2007; 7:678–689. DOI: 10.1038/nri2156

[16] Kolaczkowska E, Kubes P: Neutrophil recruitment and function in health and inflammation. Nat. Rev. Immunol. 2013; 13:159–175. DOI: 10.1038/nri3399

[17] Eskan MA, Jotwani R, Abe T, Chmelar J, Lim JH, Liang S, Ciero PA, Krauss JL, Li F, Rauner M *et al*: The leukocyte integrin antagonist Del-1 inhibits IL-17-mediated inflammatory bone loss. Nat. Immunol. 2012; 13:465–473. DOI: 10.1038/ni.2260.

[18] Kennedy AD, DeLeo FR: Neutrophil apoptosis and the resolution of infection. Immunol. Res. 2009; 43:25–61. DOI: 10.1007/s12026-008-8049-6

[19] Martin C, Burdon PC, Bridger G, Gutierrez-Ramos JC, Williams TJ, Rankin SM: Chemokines acting via CXCR2 and CXCR4 control the release of neutrophils from the bone marrow and their return following senescence. Immunity 2003; 19:583–593.

[20] Stark MA, Huo Y, Burcin TL, Morris MA, Olson TS, Ley K: Phagocytosis of apoptotic neutrophils regulates granulopoiesis via IL-23 and IL-17. Immunity 2005; 22:285–294. DOI: 10.1016/j.immuni.2005.01.011

[21] Altznauer F, Martinelli S, Yousefi S, Thürig C, Schmid I, Conway EM, Schöni MH, Vogt P, Mueller C, Fey MF *et al*: Inflammation-associated cell cycle-independent block of apoptosis by survivin in terminally differentiated neutrophils. J. Exp. Med. 2004 199:1343–1354. DOI: 10.1084/jem.20032033

[22] Belkaid Y, Naik S: Compartmentalized and systemic control of tissue immunity by commensals. Nat. Immunol. 2013 14:646–653. DOI: 10.1038/ni.2604

[23] Belkaid Y: Tailored immunity at mucosae. Immunol. Rev. 2014; 260:5–7. DOI: 10.1111/imr.12197

[24] Curtis MA, Zenobia C, Darveau RP: The relationship of the oral microbiotia to periodontal health and disease. Cell Host Microbe 2011 10:302–306. DOI: 10.1016/j.chom.2011.09.008

[25] Pham CT: Neutrophil serine proteases: specific regulators of inflammation. Nat. Rev. Immunol. 2006 6:541–550. DOI: 10.1038/nri1841

[26] Faurschou M, Borregaard N: Neutrophil granules and secretory vesicles in inflammation. Microbes Infect. 2003; 5:1317–1327.

[27] Sengeløv H, Follin P, Kjeldsen L, Lollike K, Dahlgren CNB: Mobilization of granules and secretory vesicles during in vivo exudation of human neutrophils. J. Immunol. 1995; 154:4157–4165.

[28] Sengeløv H, Kjeldsen L, Borregaard N: Control of exocytosis in early neutrophil activation. J. Immunol. 1993; 150:1535–1543.

[29] Zenobia C, Luo XL, Hashim A, Abe T, Jin L, Chang Y, Jin ZC, Sun JX, Hajishengallis G, Curtis MA *et al*: Commensal bacteria-dependent select expression of CXCL2 contributes to periodontal tissue homeostasis. Cell. Microbiol. 2013 15:1419–1426. DOI: 10.1111/cmi.12127

[30] Matute JD, Arias AA, Wright NA, Wrobel I, Waterhouse CC, Li XJ, Marchal CC, Stull ND, Lewis DB, Steele M *et al*: A new genetic subgroup of chronic granulomatous disease with autosomal recessive mutations in p40 phox and selective defects in neutrophil NADPH oxidase activity. Blood 2009; 114:3309–3315. DOI: 10.1182/blood-2009-07-231498

[31] Soler-Palacín P, Margareto C, Llobet P, Asensio O, Hernández M, Caragol I, Español T: Chronic granulomatous disease in pediatric patients: 25 years of experience. Allergol. Immunopathol. 2007; 35:83–89.

[32] Lindhe J, Lang NP, Kariing T: Clinical Periodontology and Implant Dentistry. Vol. 1, Fifth edition. Oxford: Blackwell Munksgaard; 2008.

[33] Zhang D, Chen G, Manwani D, Mortha A, Xu C, Faith JJ, Burk RD, Kunisaki Y, Jang JE, Scheiermann C *et al*: Neutrophil ageing is regulated by the microbiome. Nature 2015; 525:528–532. DOI: 10.1038/nature15367

[34] Sørensen OE, Clemmensen SN, Dahl SL, Østergaard O, Heegaard NH, Glenthøj A, Nielsen FC, Borregaard N: Papillon-Lefèvre syndrome patient reveals species-dependent requirements for neutrophil defenses. J. Clin. Invest. 2014; 124:4539–4548. DOI: 10.1172/JCI76009

[35] Roberts H, White P, Dias I, McKaig S, Veeramachaneni R, Thakker N, Grant M, Chapple I: Characterization of neutrophil function in Papillon-Lefèvre syndrome. J. Leukoc. Biol. 2016; 100:433–444. DOI: 10.1189/jlb.5A1015-489R

[36] Perera NC, Wiesmüller KH, Larsen MT, Schacher B, Eickholz P, Borregaard N, Jenne DE: NSP4 is stored in azurophil granules and released by activated neutrophils as active endoprotease with restricted specificity. J. Immunol. 2013; 191:2700–2707. DOI: 10.4049/jimmunol.1301293

[37] Uriarte SM, Edmisson JS, Jimenez-Flores E: Human neutrophils and oral microbiota: a constant tug-of-war between a harmonious and a discordant coexistence. Immunol. Rev. 2016; 273:282–298. DOI: 10.1111/imr.12451

[38] Eke PI, Dye BA, Wei L, Slade GD, Thornton-Evans GO, Borgnakke WS, Taylor GW, Page RC, Beck JD, Genco RJ: Update on prevalence of periodontitis in adults in the United States: NHANES 2009 to 2012. J. Periodontol. 2015; 86:611–622. DOI: 10.1902/jop.2015.140520

[39] Zadeh HH, Nichols FC, Miyasaki KT: The role of the cell-mediated immune response to *Actinobacillus actinomycetemcomitans* and *Porphyromonas gingivalis* in periodontitis. Periodontol. 2000 1999; 20:239–288.

[40] Borgnakke WS: Does treatment of periodontal disease influence systemic disease? Dent. Clin. North Am. 2015 59:885–917. DOI: 10.1016/j.cden.2015.06.007

[41] Seymour GJ, Ford PJ, Cullinan MP, Leishman S, Yamazaki K: Relationship between periodontal infections and systemic disease. Clin. Microbiol. Infect. 2007; 13:3–10. DOI: 10.1111/j.1469-0691.2007.01798.x

[42] Rivera MF, Lee JY, Aneja M, Goswami V, Liu L, Velsko IM, Chukkapalli SS, Bhattacharyya I, Chen H, Lucas AR *et al*: Polymicrobial infection with major periodontal pathogens induced periodontal disease and aortic atherosclerosis in hyperlipidemic ApoE(null) mice. PLoS One 2013; 8:e57178. DOI: 10.1371/journal.pone.0057178

[43] Daniel R, Gokulanathan S, Shanmugasundaram N, Lakshmigandhan M, Kavin T: Diabetes and periodontal disease. J. Pharm. Bioallied Sci. 2012 4:S280–S282. DOI: 10.4103/0975-7406.100251

[44] Lakschevitz F, Aboodi G, Tenenbaum H, Glogauer M: Diabetes and periodontal diseases: interplay and links. Curr. Diabetes Rev. 2011; 7:433–439.

[45] Lamster IB, Pagan M: Periodontal disease and the metabolic syndrome. Int. Dent. J. 2016; 9. DOI: 10.1111/idj.12264

[46] Dababneh R, Al-Wahadneh AM, Hamadneh S, Khouri A, Bissada NF: Periodontal manifestation of leukocyte adhesion deficiency type I. J. Periodontol. 2008; 79:764–768. DOI: 10.1902/jop.2008.070323

[47] Moutsopoulos NM, Konkel J, Sarmadi M, Eskan MA, Wild T, Dutzan N, Abusleme L, Zenobia C, Hosur KB, Abe T *et al*: Defective neutrophil recruitment in leukocyte adhesion deficiency type I disease causes local IL-17-driven inflammatory bone loss. Sci. Transl. Med. 2014; 6:229ra240. DOI: 10.1126/scitranslmed.3007696

[48] Ryder MI: Comparison of neutrophil functions in aggressive and chronic periodontitis. Periodontol. 2000 2010; 53:124–137. DOI: 10.1111/j.1600-0757.2009.00327.x

[49] Aboodi GM, Goldberg MB, Glogauer M: Refractory periodontitis population characterized by a hyperactive oral neutrophil phenotype. J. Periodontol. 2011; 82:726–733. DOI: 10.1902/jop.2010.100508

[50] Choi EY, Chavakis E, Czabanka MA, Langer HF, Fraemohs L, Economopoulou M, Kundu RK, Orlandi A, Zheng YY, Prieto DA *et al*: Del-1, an endogenous leukocyte-endothelial adhesion inhibitor, limits inflammatory cell recruitment. Science 2008; 322:1101–1104. DOI: 10.1126/science.1165218

[51] Berezow AB, Darveau RP: Microbial shift and periodontitis. Periodontol. 2000 2011 55:36–47. DOI: 10.1111/j.1600-0757.2010.00350.x

[52] Griffen AL, Beall CJ, Firestone ND, Gross EL, Difranco JM, Hardman JH, Vriesendorp B, Faust RA, Janies DA, Leys EJ: CORE: a phylogenetically-curated 16S rDNA database of the core oral microbiome. PLoS One 2011 6:e19051. DOI: 10.1371/journal.pone.0019051

[53] Dewhirst FE, Chen T, Izard J, Paster BJ, Tanner AC, Yu WH, Lakshmanan A, Wade WG: The human oral microbiome. J. Bacteriol. 2010; 192:5002–5017. DOI: 10.1128/JB.00542-10

[54] Wade WG: Has the use of molecular methods for the characterization of the human oral microbiome changed our understanding of the role of bacteria in the pathogenesis of periodontal disease? J. Clin. Periodontol. 2011; 38:7–16. DOI: 10.1111/j.1600-051X.2010.01679.x

[55] Hajishengallis GJLR: Dancing with the stars: how choreographed bacterial interactions dictate nososymbiocity and give rise to keystone pathogens, accessory pathogens, and pathobionts. Trends Microbiol. 2016; 24:477–489. DOI: 10.1016/j.tim.2016.02.010

[56] Socransky SS, Haffajee AD, Cugini MA, Smith C, Kent RL: Microbial complexes in subgingival plaque. J. Clin. Periodontol. 1998; 25:134–144.

[57] Costalonga M, Herzberg MC: The oral microbiome and the immunobiology of periodontal disease and caries. Immunol. Lett. 2014 162:22–38. DOI: 10.1016/j.imlet.2014.08.017

[58] Hirschfeld J: Dynamic interactions of neutrophils and biofilms. J. Oral. Microbiol. 2014; 6:26102. DOI: 10.3402/jom.v6.26102

[59] Jensen PØ, Bjarnsholt T, Phipps R, Rasmussen TB, Calum H, Christoffersen L, Moser C, Williams P, Pressler T, Givskov M *et al*: Rapid necrotic killing of polymorphonuclear leukocytes is caused by quorum-sensing-controlled production of rhamnolipid by *Pseudomonas aeruginosa*. Microbiology 2007; 153:1329–1338. DOI: 10.1099/mic.0.2006/003863-0

[60] Bjarnsholt T, Jensen PØ, Burmølle M, Hentzer M, Haagensen JA, Hougen HP, Calum H, Madsen KG, Moser C, Molin S *et al*: *Pseudomonas aeruginosa* tolerance to tobramycin, hydrogen peroxide and polymorphonuclear leukocytes is quorum-sensing dependent. Microbiology 2005; 151:373–383. DOI: 10.1099/mic.0.27463-0

[61] Claesson R, Johansson A, Belibasakis G, Hänström L, Kalfas S: Release and activation of matrix metalloproteinase 8 from human neutrophils triggered by the leukotoxin of *Actinobacillus actinomycetemcomitans*. J. Periodontal. Res. 2002; 37:353–359.

[62] Johansson A, Claesson R, Belibasakis G, Makoveichuk E, Hänström L, Olivecrona G, Sandström G, Kalfas S: Protease inhibitors, the responsible components for the serum-dependent enhancement of *Actinobacillus actinomycetemcomitans* leukotoxicity. Eur. J. Oral Sci. 2001; 109:335–341.

[63] Anwar S, Prince LR, Foster SJ, Whyte MK, Sabroe I: The rise and rise of *Staphylococcus aureus*: laughing in the face of granulocytes. Clin. Exp. Immunol. 2009; 157:216–224. DOI: 10.1111/j.1365-2249.2009.03950.x

[64] Papo N, Shai Y: A molecular mechanism for lipopolysaccharide protection of Gram-negative bacteria from antimicrobial peptides. J. Biol. Chem. 2005; 280:10378–10387. DOI: 10.1074/jbc.M412865200

[65] Yamanaka T, Furukawa T, Matsumoto-Mashimo C, Yamane K, Sugimori C, Nambu T, Mori N, Nishikawa H, Walker CB, Leung KP *et al*: Gene expression profile and pathogenicity of biofilm-forming *Prevotella intermedia* strain 17. BMC Microbiol. 2009; 9:99. DOI: 10.1186/1471-2180-9-11

[66] Gresham HD, Lowrance JH, Caver TE, Wilson BS, Cheung AL, Lindberg FP: Survival of *Staphylococcus aureus* inside neutrophils contributes to infection. J. Immunol. 2000; 164:3712–3722.

[67] Mydel P, Takahashi Y, Yumoto H, Sztukowska M, Kubica M, Gibson FCr, Kurtz DMJ, Travis J, Collins LV, Nguyen KA *et al*: Roles of the host oxidative immune response and bacterial antioxidant rubrerythrin during *Porphyromonas gingivalis* infection. PLoS Pathog. 2006; 2:e76. DOI: 10.1371/journal.ppat.0020076

[68] Tamura M, Tokuda M, Nagaoka S, Takada H: Lipopolysaccharides of *Bacteroides intermedius* (Prevotella intermedia) and Bacteroides (Porphyromonas) gingivalis induce interleukin-8 gene expression in human gingival fibroblast cultures. Infect. Immun. 1992; 11:4932–4937.

[69] Belibasakis GN, Thurnheer T, Bostanci N: Interleukin-8 responses of multi-layer gingival epithelia to subgingival biofilms: role of the "red complex" species. PLoS One 2013; 8:e81581. DOI: 10.1371/journal.pone.0081581

[70] Amin M, Grove DA, Kapus A, Glogauer M, Ellen RP: An actin-stabilizing peptide conjugate deduced from the major outer sheath protein of the bacterium *Treponema denticola*. Cell Motil. Cytoskeleton 2007; 64:662–674. DOI: 10.1002/cm.20213

[71] Lukac J, Mravak-Stipetić M, Knezević M, Vrcek J, Sistig S, Ledinsky M, Kusić Z: Phagocytic functions of salivary neutrophils in oral mucous membrane diseases. J. Oral Pathol. Med. 2003; 32:271–274.

[72] Takubo T, Yamane T, Tsuda I, Tagawa S, Tatsumi N: Polymorphonuclear neutrophils in saliva and blood: a comparative study of morphology, function and phenotype. Br. J. Biomed. Sci. 1997 54:260–266.

[73] Hajishengallis G, Maekawa T, Abe T, Hajishengallis E, Lambris JD: Complement involvement in periodontitis: molecular mechanisms and rational therapeutic approaches. Adv. Exp. Med. Biol. 2015; 865:57–74. DOI: 10.1007/978-3-319-18603-0_4

[74] Maekawa T, Abe T, Hajishengallis E, Hosur KB, DeAngelis RA, Ricklin D, Lambris JD, Hajishengallis G: Genetic and intervention studies implicating complement C3 as a major target for the treatment of periodontitis. J. Immunol. 2014; 192:6020–6027. DOI: 10.4049/jimmunol.1400569

[75] Shin J, Maekawa T, Abe T, Hajishengallis E, Hosur K, Pyaram K, Mitroulis I, Chavakis T, Hajishengallis G: DEL-1 restrains osteoclastogenesis and inhibits inflammatory bone loss in nonhuman primates. Sci. Transl. Med. 2015; 7:307ra155. DOI: 10.1126/scitranslmed.aac5380

Chapter 5

Neutrophils in Rheumatoid Arthritis: A Target for Discovering New Therapies Based on Natural Products

Elaine Cruz Rosas, Luana Barbosa Correa and
Maria das Graças Henriques

Additional information is available at the end of the chapter

http://dx.doi.org/10.5772/intechopen.68617

Abstract

Rheumatoid arthritis (RA) is a systemic autoimmune disorder with an important inflammatory component in joints. Neutrophils are the most abundant leukocytes in inflamed joints, and play an essential role in the initiation and progression of RA. Neutrophil effector mechanisms include the release of proinflammatory cytokines, reactive oxygen and nitrogen species (ROS and RNS), and granules containing degradative enzymes, which can cause further damage to the tissue and amplify the neutrophil response. Therefore, the modulation of neutrophil migration and functions is a potential target for pharmacological intervention in arthritis. The pharmacologic treatment options for RA are diverse. The current treatments are mostly symptomatic and have side effects, high costs, and an increased risk of malignancies. Because of these limitations, there is a growing interest in the use of natural products as therapies or adjunct therapies. Herbal products have attracted considerable interest over the past decade because of their multiple beneficial effects such as their antioxidant, anti-inflammatory, antiproliferative, and immunomodulatory properties. This chapter focuses on the role of neutrophils in the pathogenesis of arthritis and the action of substances from natural products as putative antirheumatic therapies.

Keywords: neutrophils, rheumatoid arthritis, herbal products, polyphenols, flavonoids, tetranortriterpenoids, inflammation

1. Introduction

Arthritis is an inflammatory joint disorder that can cause edema, pain, and loss of function. The most common types of arthritis are osteoarthritis, gout, and rheumatoid arthritis [1, 2]. Rheumatoid arthritis is a systemic, autoimmune disorder with an important inflammatory component in which genetic and environmental risk factors contribute to disease development. Its prevalence in the world population is between 0.3 and 1%, and it affects three times more women than men [3, 4].

The pathophysiology of RA is complex and appears to be initiated when the adaptive immune system (cellular or humoral) recognizes self-joint antigens as non-self, which triggers a variety of distinct inflammatory effector mechanisms, including the recruitment of leukocytes [5–8].

RA is characterized by intense inflammatory processes and joint damage that are mediated by the influx of immune system cells to the synovial space such as neutrophils, macrophages, and lymphocytes [1, 2]. A critical factor that contributes to tissue damage is the excessive production of inflammatory mediators by resident and/or infiltrated cells. Among the primary mediators involved in joint damage are free radicals, enzymes that degrade the matrix, and pro-inflammatory cytokines, including tumor necrosis factor (TNF)-α, interleukin (IL)-6 and IL-1β, as well as chemokines such as CXCL-8, lipid mediators, such as leukotriene B_4 (LTB_4) [9, 10], and endothelin (ET) [11, 12]. Inflamed synovial tissue is invasive and called pannus, which can be formed by synovial cell proliferation, angiogenesis, and the accumulation of macrophages, lymphocytes, and neutrophils [13].

Neutrophils are crucial cells that have significant roles in diverse inflammatory diseases, including acute, chronic, autoimmune, infectious, and non-infectious conditions [14]. The most well-known effector function of neutrophils is their role in innate immunity. However, recent studies have identified neutrophils as active cells during adaptive immunity, facilitating the recruitment and activation of antigen-presenting cells or directly interacting with T cells. Neutrophils are the most abundant leukocytes in inflamed joints, and the importance of these cells in the initiation and progression of human RA as well as in murine models has been demonstrated [15–18]. Therefore, neutrophils play an essential role in joint inflammation, and the modulation of neutrophil functions is considered a potential target for pharmacological intervention in arthritis [19–21].

The pharmacologic treatment options for arthritis are diverse. The current treatments are mostly symptomatic and include non-steroidal anti-inflammatory drugs (NSAIDs), corticosteroids, disease-modifying antirheumatic drugs (DMARDs), and biologic therapies. High costs and an increased risk of malignancies limit the use of these agents, in addition to the potential side effects that all therapies possess. Plant-derived products, such as polyphenols, sesquiterpenes, flavonoids, and tetranortriterpenoids, which are herbal metabolites with anti-inflammatory activity, may provide new therapeutic agents and cost-effective treatments [22, 23]. This chapter focuses on the role of neutrophils in the pathogenesis of arthritis and the action of substances from natural products as putative antirheumatic therapies.

2. Role of neutrophils in rheumatoid arthritis

2.1. Neutrophil trafficking from blood to the synovial cavity

Neutrophil recruitment is an important stage in the inflammatory development process, including autoimmune diseases such as RA. Among the circulating cells, neutrophils are the first ones to reach the synovium and are the most abundant cells in the synovial fluid [24]. In this section,

http://dx.doi.org/10.5772/intechopen.68617

we discuss the cascade of events that culminates in neutrophil entry into inflamed joints. The leukocyte recruitment cascade involves the following commonly recognized steps: capture, rolling, firm adhesion, and finally transendothelial migration.

Neutrophil release from the bone marrow to the circulating blood occurs immediately after the first signal of inflammation, serving to increase the number of neutrophils available for recruitment into the tissue in response to inflammation [25]. The mobilization of neutrophils from the bone marrow is orchestrated by the hematopoietic cytokine granulocyte colony-stimulating factor (G-CSF). G-CSF mobilizes neutrophils indirectly by shifting the balance between CXCR4 and CXCR2 ligands [26]. In response to the release of inflammatory mediators such as TNF-α and IL-17, the adjacent vascular endothelium becomes activated. Cell surface proteins of the selectin family termed E- and P-selectin and their ligands (L-selectin) mediate this initial neutrophil capture. Neutrophil rolling through the endothelium facilitates their contact with chemotactic factors that promotes neutrophil activation [27]. Chemokines (CXCR-1 or 2 ligands, such as IL-8), the C5a fragment of the complement system, and leukotriene B_4 (LTB_4) are responsible for neutrophil mobilization to the synovial fluid [28–30].

Firm adhesion is mediated by interactions between β_2 integrins (LFA-1, CD11a/CD18, and MAC-1, CD11b/CD18) and their ligand (ICAM-1). Integrins are usually in an inactive state on neutrophil and become activated after the triggering of G protein-coupled receptors such as chemokine receptors [31]. The binding of integrins to their ligands activates signaling pathways in neutrophils stabilizing adhesion and initiating cell motility [32, 33]. This signaling also regulates actin polymerization, which controls the direction of neutrophil movement [34, 35]. The final stage in the adhesion cascade is the ultimate migration of the neutrophil from the vasculature into the inflamed tissue. Passage through the endothelial cell layer occurs both paracellularly (between endothelial cells) and by a transcellular route (over the endothelial cell). Paracellular migration of neutrophils is mediated by binding to endothelial proteins that target neutrophils to intercellular junctions and facilitate their passage through them. To reach the inflamed joint, neutrophils must pass over the basal membrane, which occurs through the degradation of extracellular matrix molecules by proteases stored inside the cells, such as matrix metalloproteinases (MMPs) and serine proteases [14].

In inflammatory foci, neutrophils find immune complexes on the synovium that bind to Fcγ receptors on the neutrophil membrane, triggering their degranulation and reactive oxygen species (ROS) production [36]. In RA pathology, oxidative stress is a result of inadequate ROS release by neutrophils [37]. Oxygen radicals cause DNA damage and oxidation of lipids, proteins, and lipoproteins and may be involved in immunoglobulin mutations that lead to rheumatoid factor (RF) formation [38, 39]. Moreover, proteins from neutrophil degranulation are found at high concentrations in the RA synovial fluid and could be responsible for cartilage and tissue damage, activation of cytokines and soluble receptors, inhibition of chondrocyte proliferation and activation of synoviocytes proliferation and invasion [40–43]. In addition, activated neutrophils also generate chemoattractants (such as IL-8 and LTB_4) that promote further neutrophil recruitment and amplify the inflammatory response (see **Figure 1**).

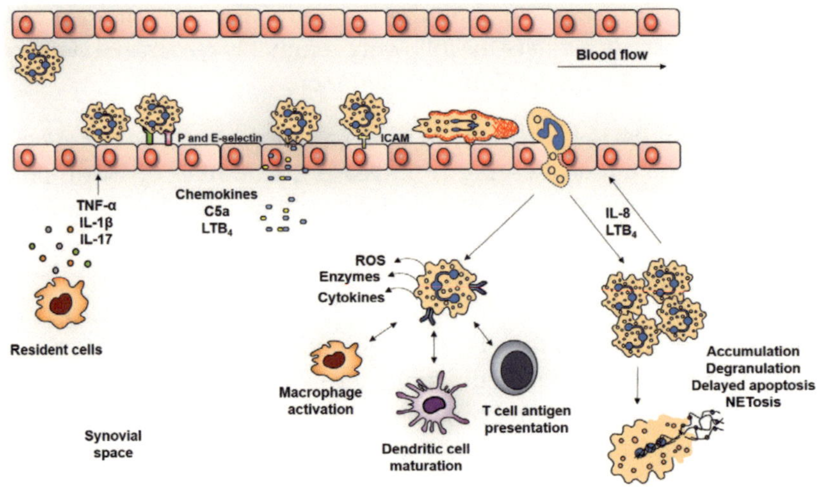

Figure 1. Overview of the role of neutrophils in arthritis. Neutrophils leave blood vessels after chemotactic signals from inflamed tissues that promote the firm adhesion of neutrophils to endothelial cells mediated by adhesion molecules, which induce neutrophil activation and actin filament formation followed by transendothelial migration toward the inflammatory foci. Immune complexes and proinflammatory molecules activate neutrophils, which then produce ROS and release enzymes responsible for cartilage destruction. Activated neutrophils communicate with other cells of the immune system through the secretion of cytokines and chemokines and by antigen presentation in conjunction with MHC class II. Neutrophils can undergo a special form of cell death called NETosis. This results in the release of a complex of nuclear and granule molecules called NETs contributing to tissue damage. Activated neutrophils also generate chemoattractants (such as IL-8 and LTB_4), forming a positive-feedback loop that promotes further neutrophil recruitment and amplifies the acute inflammatory response. Finally, effective neutrophil apoptosis is required for the resolution of inflammation. However, delayed neutrophil apoptosis occurs in the inflamed joint, which results in persistent inflammation and tissue damage due to the continued release of ROS, granule enzymes, and cytokines.

2.2. Neutrophil action in rheumatoid arthritis

Neutrophils are key cells in articular inflammation that are abundant in the synovial fluid and pannus of patients with active RA [44], a typical knee joint may have 2×10^9 cells, of which 90% are neutrophils [24]. These cells are mobilized to synovial tissue by chemoattractant mediators, such as CXCL1, CXCL2, endothelin (ET)-1, and leukotriene B_4, a process in which resident macrophages play a central role [11, 45, 46].

For many years, the major contribution of neutrophils to the pathology of RA was thought to be their cytotoxic potential, since neutrophils participate in the pathogenesis of arthritis by promoting the inflammatory process and cartilage degradation, as well as bone resorption. However, neutrophils are now recognized to have an active role in orchestrating the progression of inflammation through regulating the functions of other immune cells [47, 48], and current research has shown that these cells are involved in RA onset [49, 50].

In the synovial cavity, activated neutrophils exhibit an increased expression of plasma membrane receptors such as major histocompatibility complex (MHC) class II molecules and present antigens to T lymphocytes, an immune function that they share with macrophages and dendritic cells (DCs) [51]. In addition, the interaction of neutrophils with other cells induces the secretion of MMP-8 and MMP-9, and a repertoire of cytokines (IL-1β, IL-12, IL-18, IL-23, and TNF-α) and chemokines (CCL-2, CCL-4, CCL-5, and CXCL-8), including TNF ligand superfamily member (RANKL) [52, 53] and TNFSF13B (also known as BLyS or BAFF) [54], which are implicated in the activation of osteoclasts and B lymphocytes, respectively, regulate the function of other immune cells [48, 55–57].

Neutrophils from patients with RA are functionally very different from those isolated from healthy individuals. RA blood neutrophils are already primed for ROS production [58] and striking differences in gene and protein expression exist between peripheral blood neutrophils from patients with RA and their healthy counterparts [18], including higher levels of membrane-expressed TNF and myeloblastin (also known as PR-3 or cANCA antigen) in RA [59].

In RA patients, neutrophils can be activated by immune complexes, such as RF or anti-citrullinated protein antibodies (ACPAs), both within the synovial fluid and deposited on the articular cartilage surface [60]. These complexes engage Fcγ receptors and thereby trigger neutrophil activation, which release ROS and RNS [61, 62], collagenases, gelatinases, neutrophil myeloperoxidase (MPO), elastase, and cathepsin G into the synovial fluid and joints [14, 55, 56, 63] due to frustrated phagocytosis [60].

2.2.1. *Pain in rheumatoid arthritis and neutrophils*

One of the most prevalent symptoms of RA is the increase in sensitivity to joint pain (hyperalgesia), which causes movement limitations. Despite its clinical relevance, strategies for the treatment of arthralgia remain limited. In animal models, hyperalgesia (inflammatory pain) is defined as hypernociception (a decreased nociceptive threshold) [64]. It is broadly accepted that articular hypernociception results mainly from the direct and indirect effects of inflammatory mediators on the sensitization (increased excitability) of primary nociceptive fibers that innervate the inflamed joints [65–67]. Prostaglandins and sympathetic amines are the key mediators of this process. Furthermore, other mediators, such as the cytokines TNF-α, IL-1β, IL-6, and IL-17 play a crucial role in the pathogenesis of arthritis, increasing the recruitment of neutrophils into the joint and driving the enhanced production of chemokines and degradative enzymes [68–70]. In addition, endothelin-1 (ET-1), acting directly or indirectly, also sensitizes primary nociceptive neurons [71–74].

During the inflammatory process, the migrating neutrophils participate in the cascade of events leading to mechanical hypernociception, by mediating the release of hyperalgesic molecules (such as MPO, MMPs, hypochlorite, superoxide anion, and PGE_2) capable of activating nociceptive neurons and causing pain [17, 75–78].

Indeed, decreased inflammation and joint destruction have been directly correlated with reduced neutrophil influx into the joints, as observed in mouse models by means of antibody blockade or the gene deletion of chemoattractant receptors such as CXCR1, CXCR2, and BLT1 (LTB_4 receptor) [15, 79]. Therefore, the blockade of neutrophil migration could be a target in the development of new analgesic drugs [77].

2.2.2. *Citrullinated autoantigens and NETs in rheumatoid arthritis*

Citrullination is the natural posttranslational conversion of arginine to citrulline mediated by peptidyl arginine deiminases (PADs), enzymes present in macrophages, dendritic cells, and neutrophils. Experimental evidence indicates that citrullination is involved in the breakdown of immune tolerance and may generate neoantigens (neoAgs) that become additional targets during epitope spreading [80]. Citrullinated residues stimulate the production of anti-citrullinated protein antibodies (ACPAs) in predisposed individuals. It has been observed that ACPAs can be present for several years before any clinical signs of arthritis appear [81–83]. A substantial increase in the number and titer of many antibodies against posttranslationally modified proteins is also seen shortly before the onset of arthritis. Citrullinated Ags have increased immunogenicity and arthritogenicity, and their presence in arthritic joints correlates with disease severity [80, 84–86].

Osteoclasts are dependent on citrullinating enzymes for their normal maturation and display citrullinated antigens on their cell surface in a non-inflamed state. In humans, the binding of ACPAs to osteoclasts in the bone compartment induces IL-8 secretion. In turn, IL-8 sensitizes and/or activates sensory neurons by binding to CXC chemokine receptor (CXCR) 1 and CXCR2 on peripheral nociceptors [87–90], producing IL 8 dependent joint pain that is associated with ACPA-mediated bone loss.

IL-8 release contributes to the chemoattraction of neutrophils [49], which play critical roles in initiating and maintaining joint-inflammatory processes that have been described in experimental arthritis [36, 91]. However, the exact roles that neutrophils play in the posttranslational modification of proteins and disease initiation and progression in RA remain unclear. Recent evidence suggests that, among the various mechanisms by which neutrophils cause tissue damage and promote autoimmunity, aberrant formation of neutrophil extracellular traps (NETs) could play important roles in the pathogenesis of RA [50].

NETs are released during a process of cellular death named NETosis. NETosis occurs with neutrophils upon contact with bacteria, fungi [92], or under several inflammatory stimuli. This process is associated with changes in the morphology of the cells, which eventually lead to cell death with extrusion of NETs [93, 94]. This process requires calcium mobilization, reactive oxygen species (ROS) produced by NADPH oxidase, neutrophil chromatin decondensation mediated by neutrophil elastase (NE) and myeloperoxidase (MPO), and chromatin modification via the citrullination of histones by peptidyl arginine deiminase 4 (PAD4) [95–99]. NETs are a network of extracellular fibers, which contain nuclear compounds as DNA and histones and that are covered with antimicrobial enzymes and granular components, such as MPO, NE, cathepsin G, and other microbicidal peptides [93, 94]. In the extracellular environment, NET fibers entrap microorganisms, and their enzymes and granular substances reach locally high concentrations and are thus able to cleave virulence factors and kill microorganisms [95, 100, 101].

Although NETs play a key role in the defense against pathogens, they may cause undesirable effects to the host, which has increased the interest in the role of neutrophils and NETs in autoimmunity. Augmented NET formation was first described in preeclampsia and ANCA-associated vasculitis and followed by the description in a series of autoimmune conditions, including psoriasis, systemic lupus erythematosus (SLE), antiphospholipid antibody syndrome (APS), and RA [50, 100, 102–105]. Neutrophil extracellular traps are an obvious source of nuclear material. Among these are a range of cytoplasmic and extracellular citrullinated antigens, well-established targets of the ACPAs found in RA [50, 100]. The protein contents of NETs not only serve as targets for autoantibody and immune complex formation but also induce further NETosis, resulting in a harmful positive-feedback loop. These factors form an inflammatory microenvironment that may trigger a strong autoimmune response in individuals with the corresponding susceptibility [106, 107]. Pro-inflammatory cytokines, such as TNF-α and IL-17, as well as autoantibodies stimulate the formation of NETs and affect their protein composition [50]. Additionally, NETs have been shown to stimulate autoimmunity via the production of interferons and activation of the complement cascade. Interferons activate both the innate and adaptive immune systems, inducing a Th1 immune response and stimulating B cells toward the generation of autoantibodies [108]. The deposition of NETs observed in various inflammatory pathologies is associated with the circulating cell-free DNA (cfDNA) levels in biological fluids, such as plasma and serum, from patients [100, 101, 109]. Therefore, circulatory cfDNA could eventually be utilized as a marker of NETs in these pathologies, while the determination of the DNA levels might facilitate the monitoring of disease activity and assessment of the effectiveness of a selected therapeutic strategy.

Neutrophils have been traditionally viewed as short-lived cells that die at sites of inflammation; however, some evidence suggests that they can prolong their life span upon specific stimuli and transmigrate away from inflammatory loci [48, 110, 111]. Conditions within the synovial joint, such as hypoxia [112] and the presence of antiapoptotic cytokines (including TNF, granulocyte-macrophage colony-stimulating factor (GM CSF), and IL 8) [113, 114], can increase neutrophil survival for up to several days [115, 116], which contributes to enhanced tissue damage.

As described above, neutrophils play an essential role on innate and adaptive immunity in RA physiopathology, contributing to tissue lesions in RA, and therefore represent a promising pharmacological target in RA. Pharmacological strategies that inhibit or reduce neutrophil mobilization or activation could be successful in RA treatment.

3. Neutrophils as therapeutic targets

Animal models have been extensively used in studies of RA pathogenesis. Despite the inherent limitations of all animal models, several rodent models have greatly contributed to the overall knowledge of important processes/mediators in the generation of inflammation, cartilage destruction, and bone resorption. In addition, the pharmaceutical industry has used these models for testing potential anti-arthritic agents, leading to important advances in therapeutic interventions for this destructive disease [117]. Such models include collagen-induced arthritis, collagen antibody-induced arthritis, zymosan-induced arthritis, the methylated BSA model, and genetically manipulated or spontaneous arthritis models such as the TNF-α-transgenic mouse, K/BxN mouse, and Skg mouse [118]. Many of these models show that neutrophils are the first immune cells to enter the arthritic joint, and that early measures of joint inflammation correlate with neutrophil infiltration [45, 119, 120]. In this section, we highlight pharmacological approaches targeting neutrophil recruitment and activity, which present a therapeutic benefit to patients with RA.

The current treatments available to RA patients include glucocorticoids, non-steroidal anti-inflammatory drugs, and disease-modifying antirheumatic drugs. Only disease-modifying agents—and to some extent glucocorticoids—can impede or halt the inflammatory and destructive disease processes [121]. With a more complete understanding of the immune-inflammatory events that occur in the pathogenesis of RA, scientists have developed therapeutic strategies that include monoclonal antibodies and receptor constructs, which target specific soluble or cell-surface molecules of interest. Biological agents such as monoclonal antibodies and recombinant proteins that target TNF-α, CD20, CTLA-4 (cytotoxic T-lymphocyte-associated protein 4), and the IL-1 receptor as well as therapies based on the blockade of T-cell and B-cell functions have shown efficacy in controlling the physical signs and pain associated with RA [122, 123].

Many interventions used to treat RA exert inhibitory effects on neutrophil responses in inflammation. However, non-steroid anti-inflammatory drugs (NSAIDS), DMARDs, and biologics do not specifically target neutrophil function [124].

Most NSAIDs inhibit the action of the cyclo-oxygenase-1 and -2 (COX-1 and -2) enzymes, which metabolize arachidonic acid into inflammatory mediators of the prostaglandin family. NSAIDs have been shown to inhibit neutrophil adherence, decrease degranulation and oxidant production, inhibit neutrophil elastase activity, and induce neutrophil apoptosis [125–127]. Corticosteroids induce anti-inflammatory signals by several mechanisms; a major one may be to reduce the expression of cytokine-induced genes. They enter all cells and bind to the cytoplasmic steroid receptor, and then this complex translocates to the nucleus where it is recognized by specific DNA sequences. The major effect of binding to DNA is the suppression of transcription by opposing the activation of the transcription factors AP-1 and NF-κB [128]. Corticosteroids have been shown to inhibit neutrophil degranulation and ROS production, decrease production of inflammatory mediators, and prevent neutrophil adhesion and migration into RA joints [44, 129–131]. The most widely used DMARD in clinic settings is methotrexate, a compound that blocks folic acid metabolism. Its benefits in RA include the stimulation of neutrophil apoptosis [116], inhibition of the NF-κB pathway [132], and reduced adhesion molecule expression and LTB_4 production [133], consequently decreasing neutrophil recruitment and ROS production [134].

Anti-TNF-α therapies are also widely used for the treatment of RA patients. TNF primes the neutrophil respiratory burst, upregulates the expression of adhesion molecules, cytokines and chemokines, and at high local concentrations can stimulate ROS production in adherent neutrophils [135–138]. Three different TNF inhibitors are available for RA patients who fail to respond adequately to standard DMARD therapy. Infliximab and adalimumab are monoclonal antibodies against TNF, whereas etanercept is a TNFRII fusion protein. All three drugs sequester soluble TNF [139]. Reports regarding the direct effect of anti-TNF agents on neutrophils have been published, and these drugs have been shown to decrease the mobilization of neutrophils from the peripheral blood to inflamed joints [140], decrease *ex vivo* neutrophil ROS production [20], and reduce neutrophil chemotactic and adhesive properties [141].

http://dx.doi.org/10.5772/intechopen.68617

Tocilizumab, a monoclonal antibody that blocks the soluble and tissue-expressed IL-6 receptor, is also proving to be a highly effective biologic agent in RA treatment [142]. Neutrophils are a major source of soluble IL-6 receptors, which they shed in large quantities when activated, and their accumulation in high numbers within the synovial joint could contribute significantly to IL-6 signaling within the synovium through trans-signaling [143]. *In vivo* therapeutic blockade of IL-6 with tocilizumab induces transient neutropenia caused by apoptosis or phagocytosis of apoptotic neutrophils but does not impair antibacterial neutrophil functions [144].

Despite the clinical efficacy of these therapies, many patients do not exhibit significant responses or discontinue treatment because of adverse effects. In addition, the limited availability of biological agents in developing countries, the need for parenteral administration of these products, and the high cost restrict access to such therapies for many RA patients worldwide, and this promotes a continuous search for new therapeutic targets and the development of new drugs [145]. Due to these limitations, interest has grown in the use of alternative treatments and herbal therapies for arthritis patients [146, 147] (**Table 1**).

Therapy	Effect on neutrophil response	Reference
Non-steroidal anti-inflammatory drugs (NSAIDS)	Inhibit neutrophil adherence, decrease neutrophil degranulation and ROS production, inhibit neutrophil elastase activity, and induce neutrophil apoptosis	[125–127]
Corticosteroids	Inhibit neutrophil degranulation and ROS production, decrease the production of inflammatory mediators, and prevent neutrophil adhesion and migration into RA joints	[44, 129–131]
Disease-modifying antirheumatic drugs (DMARDs)	Stimulate neutrophil apoptosis, inhibit the NF-κB pathway, and reduce adhesion molecule expression, LTB_4 production, neutrophil recruitment, and ROS production	[116, 132–134]
TNF-α inhibitors	Decrease neutrophil mobilization from the peripheral blood to inflamed joints and reduce *ex vivo* neutrophil ROS production and neutrophil chemotactic and adhesive properties	[20, 140, 141]
IL-6 inhibitor	Induce transient neutropenia caused by apoptosis or phagocytosis of apoptotic neutrophils but not impair antibacterial neutrophil functions	[144]

Table 1. Current therapeutic targets for arthritis and their effect on neutrophils.

4. Plant-derived molecules as emerging therapies for arthritis

Current arthritis treatments result in unwanted side effects and tend to be expensive, and natural products devoid of such disadvantages offer a novel opportunity. The use of natural products represents a promising alternative to treat rheumatic diseases, in particular by acting as therapeutic adjuvants to reduce the daily doses of conventional drugs that RA patients administer [148–150]. In this section, we highlight future perspectives in the treatment of RA with natural compounds, mainly herbal compounds, to minimize the harmful effects of the over-activation of neutrophils.

Decreased inflammation and joint destruction have been directly correlated with reduced neutrophil influx into the joints, as observed in mouse models by means of antibody blockade or the gene deletion of chemoattractant receptors such as CXCR1, CXCR2, and BLT1 (LTB_4 receptor) [15, 79]. The prospect of new drugs obtained from herbal products (or from structures of herbal products) plays a compelling role in drug discovery and development [151].

As previously mentioned, pharmacologic treatment options for arthritis are diverse and present several side effects. Furthermore, the high costs and increased risk of malignancies limit the use of such agents. Because of these limitations, there is a growing interest in the use of natural products as therapies or adjunct therapies [22]. Plant-derived products such as polyphenols, sesquiterpenes, flavonoids, and tetranortriterpenoids, which are herbal metabolites, are considered to have potential activity to block inflammation, and they may provide new therapeutic agents and cost-effective treatments [22, 23]. These natural products have attracted considerable interest over the past decade because of their multiple beneficial effects, such as their antioxidant, anti-inflammatory, antiproliferative, and immunomodulatory properties. In this section, we discuss the plant-derived products that have been most studied in RA experimental models and/or clinical trials (**Table 2**).

4.1. Quercetin

Quercetin (**Figure 2a**) is the major dietary flavonol found in fruits, vegetables, and beverages, such as tea and red wine [152]. Several epidemiological and experimental studies support the antioxidant, anti-inflammatory, antiangiogenic, antiproliferative, and proapoptotic effects of this molecule [153–155]. Preclinical studies on primary cells and animal models, as

Compound	Chemical class	Arthritis experimental model	Reference
Quercetin	Flavonoid	Adjuvant-induced arthritis	[156]
Methyl gallate	Polyphenol	Zymosan-induced arthritis	[171]
Gedunin	Tetranortriterpenoid	Zymosan-induced arthritis	[176]
Epigallocatechin gallate	Polyphenol	Collagen-induced arthritis	[179]
Curcumin	Polyphenol	Collagen-induced arthritis	[191]

Table 2. Herbal products that exhibit anti-arthritic potential in animal models.

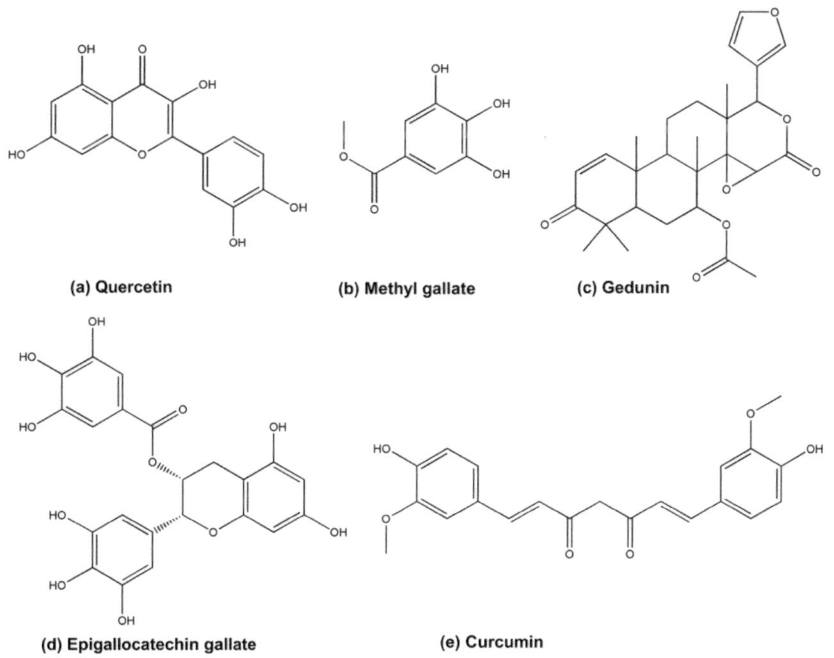

Figure 2. Chemical structure of (a) quercetin, (b) methyl gallate, (c) gedunin, (d) epigallocatechin gallate, and (e) curcumin.

well as clinical studies, suggest an inhibitory action of quercetin in RA. Quercetin has been reported to lower the levels of IL-1β, C-reactive protein, and monocyte chemotactic protein-1 (MCP-1), and restore plasma antioxidant capacity. In addition, quercetin increased the expression of hemeoxygenase-1 in the joints of arthritic rats. Finally, quercetin inhibited the twofold increase in NF-κB activity observed in joints after arthritis induction [156].

There are divergent data on the effect of quercetin in neutrophils. For instance, *in vitro*, quercetin inhibited myeloperoxidase activity [157] but had no effect on lipopolysaccharide-induced neutrophil surface expression of the adhesion molecules L-selectin (CD62L) and β2 integrin (CD11b/Mac1), [158] which are related to rolling and firm adhesion, respectively [159]. In paw edema induced by carrageen, quercetin did not inhibit the increase in myeloperoxidase, which is used as a marker of neutrophil recruitment [160]. Therefore, it seems unlikely that quercetin would inhibit neutrophil recruitment [158]. On the other hand, quercetin inhibits the fMLP-induced increase in intracellular calcium, [158] which is necessary for actin polymerization and consequently neutrophil migration [159]. In addition, *in vitro*, quercetin blocked human neutrophil mobilization through the inhibition of the cellular signaling responsible for actin polymerization in association with the down-regulation of adhesion molecules [161], indicating that treatment with this flavonoid is a conceivable approach to control excessive neutrophil recruitment during inflammation and to prevent neutrophil-mediated tissue lesions [162] (**Table 3**).

4.2. *Schinus terebinthifolius* and methyl gallate

S. terebinthifolius Raddi (Anacardiaceae) is a native plant from South America. It has been used in folk medicine as teas, infusions, or tinctures, as an anti-inflammatory, febrifuge, analgesic,

Compound	Molecular targets/mechanisms	Reference
Quercetin	Inhibits IL-1β, C-reactive protein, and MCP-1 levels. Restores plasma antioxidant capacity, increases HO-1 expression, and inhibits NF-κB activity in joints Inhibits myeloperoxidase activity in neutrophils and blocks neutrophil mobilization	[156, 157, 161]
Methyl gallate	Reduces edema formation, total leukocyte accumulation, neutrophil migration and IL-6, TNF-α, CXCL-1, IL-1β, LTB_4 and PGE_2 production in zymosan-induced arthritis. Impairs neutrophil chemotaxis and adhesion	[171]
Gedunin	Attenuates zymosan-induced articular edema, neutrophil migration, hypernociception, and the production of IL-6, TNF-α, LTB_4 and PGE_2 and prevents increases in lipid bodies. Decreases neutrophil shape changes, chemotaxis, and lipid body formation	[176]
Epigallocatechin gallate	Ameliorates the severity of arthritis and regulates the expression of cytokines, chemokines, MMPs, ROS, NO, COX-2, and PGE_2. Affects neutrophil functionality and inhibits IL-8 and MIP-3α expression	[179–184, 186–189]
Curcumin	Suppresses collagen-induced arthritis by reducing cellular infiltration, synovial hyperplasia, cartilage destruction, and bone erosion. Blocks neutrophil recruitment	[191, 193]

Table 3. Major molecular targets and anti-arthritic mechanisms of herbal products.

and depurative agent and to treat urogenital system illnesses [163]. Scientific reports demonstrated that *S. terebinthifolius* extracts and fractions are rich in polyphenols and display antioxidant, antibacterial, and antiallergic properties in different experimental models [164–166]. The HPLH chromatograms of hydroalcoholic extracts from *S. terebinthifolius* leaves (ST-70) reveal that methyl gallate (MG, **Figure 2b**) is one of the major polyphenol components of the ST-70 extract [167]. Methyl gallate has been extensively studied because of its antioxidant, antitumor, and antimicrobial activities [168–170]. Pharmacological studies have shown that ST-70 and MG also have an anti-inflammatory effect and may have potential activity against arthritis. Pretreatment with ST-70 or MG markedly reduced knee-joint thickness, total leukocyte (mainly neutrophil) infiltration, and reduced the production of inflammatory mediators associated with arthritis such as CXCL-1/KC, IL-6, TNF-α, IL-1β, LTB_4 and PGE_2. ST-70 and MG also inhibited murine neutrophil chemotaxis induced by CXCL-1/KC *in vitro*, and

MG impaired the adhesion of these cells to TNF-α-primed endothelial cells [167, 171]. These results provide some evidence that MG inhibits neutrophil activation and adhesion molecules expression and consequently prevents the neutrophil entry into inflammatory sites (**Table 3**).

Moreover, unlike potassium diclofenac, the long-term oral administration of ST-70 does not induce lethality or gastric damage in mice, which suggests that ST-70 could be used to treat inflammatory conditions such as arthritis with less toxicity [167].

4.3. *Carapa guianensis* and gedunin

C. guianensis Aublet is a member of the Meliaceae family that is widely used in folk medicine in Brazil and other countries surrounding the Amazon rainforest [172]. Anti-inflammatory and analgesic activities are among the most remarkable properties attributed by ethnopharmacological research to the oil extracted from *C. guianensis* seeds, mainly for rheumatic pain and arthritis [172, 173]. *C. guianensis* oil and six different tetranortriterpenoids (TNTP) isolated from the oil were able to significantly inhibit zymosan-induced knee joint edema formation and protein extravasation. TNTP pretreatment inhibited the increase in total leukocyte and neutrophil numbers in the synovial fluid. TNTP also impaired the production of TNF-α, IL-1β, and CXCL-8/IL-8, and significantly inhibited the expression of the NF-κB p65 subunit [174].

Gedunin (**Figure 2c**) is a natural tetranortriterpenoid isolated from vegetal species of the Meliaceae family and is known to inhibit the stress-induced chaperone heat shock protein (Hsp) 90 [175]. Mouse pretreatment and posttreatment with gedunin impaired zymosan-induced edema formation and total leukocyte influx mainly due to the inhibition of neutrophil migration and reduced articular hypernociception. Gedunin also reduced the *in situ* expression of preproET-1 mRNA and IL-6, TNF-α, LTB_4 and PGE_2 production and prevented increases in the number of lipid bodies in synovial leukocytes [176]. Lipid bodies are important sites for the synthesis and storage of lipid mediators and they increase in number during inflammatory responses [177]. In neutrophils, gedunin impaired ET-1-induced shape changes, blocked ET-1- and LTB_4-induced chemotaxis, decreased ET-1-induced lipid body formation and impaired neutrophil adhesion to TNF-α-primed endothelial cells [176]. The combined *in vitro* and *in vivo* effects of gedunin reveal its potential as an anti-arthritic candidate, especially its direct effect on key cells involved in articular inflammation such as neutrophils (**Table 3**).

4.4. Epigallocatechin gallate

Epigallocatechin gallate (EGCG, **Figure 2d**) is one of the main components of green tea [178]. It has antioxidative, anti-inflammatory, antitumor, and chemopreventive properties. The potential disease-modifying effects of green tea on arthritis have been reported; for example, in a mouse model of RA, the induction and severity of arthritis was ameliorated by the prophylactic administration of green tea polyphenols [179]. Subsequent studies suggested that EGCG possesses remarkable potential to prevent chronic diseases like OA and RA [180–184]. The anti-inflammatory and anti-arthritic effects of EGCG are supported by *in vitro* and *in vivo* data indicating that EGCG can regulate the expression of cytokines, chemokines, MMPs,

ROS, nitric oxide (NO), COX-2, and PGE_2 in cell types relevant to the pathogenesis of RA [179–184]. In *in vivo* studies, EGCG was found to inhibit inflammation in mouse models by affecting the functioning of T cells and neutrophils [185, 186]. IL-8 is the most powerful chemo-attractant for neutrophils in the target tissue. EGCG is a very effective inhibitor of IL-1β and of TNF-α-induced IL-8 and macrophage-inflammatory protein-3α (MIP-3α) expression in different cell types [187–189]. These *in vitro* and *in vivo* observations indicated the efficacy of EGCG and demonstrate that it can modulate multiple signal transduction pathways in a fashion that suppresses the expression of inflammatory mediators that play a role in the pathogenesis of arthritis (**Table 3**).

4.5. Curcumin

Curcumin (**Figure 2e**) is a yellow-colored polyphenol found in the rhizome of turmeric. It has antioxidant, anti-inflammatory, antiapoptotic, and anticarcinogenic properties [190]. Oral administration of curcumin suppressed type II collagen-induced arthritis (CIA) in mice by reducing cellular infiltration, synovial hyperplasia, cartilage destruction, and bone erosion. Moreover, the production of MMP-1 and MMP-3 was inhibited by curcumin in CIA and in TNF-α-stimulated RA fibroblast-like synoviocytes (RA-FLS) and chondrocytes [191].

In vitro, it has been reported that curcumin decreases IL-1β-induced expression of the pro-inflammatory cytokine IL-6 and vascular endothelial growth factor (VEGF) in RA-FLS [192]. In addition, curcumin blocks neutrophil recruitment through the inhibition of cellular signaling responsible for actin polymerization in association with the down-regulation of adhesion molecules [193]. It has also been shown to induce apoptosis of RA-FLS (which are resistant to apoptosis) by increasing the expression of the proapoptotic protein Bax and down-regulating the expression of the antiapoptotic protein Bcl-2 [190]. Some molecular mechanisms related to curcumin have been identified. In a human synovial fibroblast cell line (MH7A) stimulated with IL-1β, curcumin blocked the activation of the NF-κB pathway and induced deactivation of the ERK-1/2 pathway [192]. In addition, this polyphenol inhibited activating phosphorylation of protein kinase Cδ (PKCδ) in CIA, RA-FLS, and chondrocytes. Curcumin also suppressed JNK and c-Jun activation in those cells [191].

In a clinical trial with RA patients, curcumin reduced reported pain, tenderness, and swelling of joints [194]. A curcumin-based medicine, Meriva®, demonstrated efficacy in clinical trials with patients with osteoarthritis by reducing reported pain [195]. In another clinical trial, treatment with Meriva® reduced stiffness and physical signs of RA (treadmill test) along with IL-1, IL-6, and VCAM-1 production [196] (**Table 3**).

5. Conclusion

In RA, neutrophils are key cells that are recognized to play an active role in orchestrating the progress of inflammation, through the release of pro-inflammatory cytokines, ROS, RNS, and NETs, which potentially affect the activities of both neutrophils and other cell types, such as resident mononuclear cells and chondrocytes. In addition, neutrophils participate in the cascade of events leading to mechanical hypernociception. Therefore, neutrophils participate in the pathogenesis of arthritis by promoting the inflammatory process, degradation of cartilage, and bone resorption. The modulation of neutrophil migration and functions in RA can be considered a potential target for pharmacological intervention in arthritis. The pharmacologic treatment options for arthritis are diverse. High costs and an increased risk of malignancies limit the use of these agents, in addition to the potential for side effects that all therapies possess. Nevertheless, herbal metabolites with anti-inflammatory activity and inhibitory action in neutrophils may provide new therapeutic agents and cost-effective treatments.

Acknowledgements

This work was supported by Brazilian grants from Coordenadoria de Aperfeiçoamento de Pessoal de Nível Superior (CAPES), Conselho Nacional de Desenvolvimento Científico e Tecnológico (CNPq), and Fundação Carlos Chagas Filho de Amparo à Pesquisa do Estado do Rio de Janeiro (FAPERJ). L. B. Correa is a student of the post-graduation Program in Cellular and Molecular Biology from Instituto Oswaldo Cruz, FIOCRUZ, Rio de Janeiro, Brazil.

Author details

Elaine Cruz Rosas[1,2*], Luana Barbosa Correa[1,2] and Maria das Graças Henriques[1,2]

*Address all correspondence to: ecrosas@fiocruz.br

1 Laboratory of Applied Pharmacology, Farmanguinhos, Oswaldo Cruz Foundation, Rio de Janeiro, Brazil

2 National Institute of Science and Technology of Innovation on Diseases of Neglected Populations (INCT-IDPN), Rio de Janeiro, Brazil

References

[1] Wong SH, Lord JM. Factors underlying chronic inflammation in rheumatoid arthritis (in Eng). Archivum Immunologiae et Therapiae Experimentalis (Warsz). Nov-Dec 2004;**52**(6):379–388

[2] Scott DL, Wolfe F, Huizinga TW. Rheumatoid arthritis (in Eng). Lancet. Sep 2010; **376**(9746):1094–1108

[3] Helmick CG. Estimates of the prevalence of arthritis and other rheumatic conditions in the United States. Part I (in Eng). Arthritis & Rheumatology. Jan 2008;**58**(1):15–25

[4] Singh JA. 2015 American College of Rheumatology Guideline for the treatment of rheumatoid arthritis (in Eng). Arthritis & Rheumatology. Jan 2016;**68**(1):1–26

[5] Arend WP. The pathophysiology and treatment of rheumatoid arthritis (in Eng). Arthritis & Rheumatology. Apr 1997;**40**(4):595–597

[6] Issekutz AC, Meager A, Otterness I, Issekutz TB. The role of tumour necrosis factor-alpha and IL-1 in polymorphonuclear leucocyte and T lymphocyte recruitment to joint inflammation in adjuvant arthritis (in Eng). Clinical & Experimental Immunology. Jul 1994;**97**(1):26–32

[7] Kasama T, Miwa Y, Isozaki T, Odai T, Adachi M, Kunkel SL. Neutrophil-derived cytokines: potential therapeutic targets in inflammation (in Eng). Current Drug Targets—Inflammation & Allergy. Jun 2005;**4**(3):273–279

[8] Mitani Y, Honda A, Jasin HE. Polymorphonuclear leukocyte adhesion to articular cartilage is inhibited by cartilage surface macromolecules (in Eng). Rheumatology International. Jul 2001;**20**(5):180–185

[9] Maini RN, Taylor PC. Anti-cytokine therapy for rheumatoid arthritis (in Eng). Annual Review of Medicine. 2000;**51**:207–229

[10] Feldmann M, Charles P, Taylor P, Maini RN. Biological insights from clinical trials with anti-TNF therapy (in Eng). Springer Seminars in Immunopathology. 1998;**20**(1–2):211–228

[11] Conte FEP. Endothelins modulate inflammatory reaction in zymosan-induced arthritis: Participation of LTB4, TNF-alpha, and CXCL-1 (in Eng). Journal of Leukocyte Biology. Sep 2008;**84**(3):652–660

[12] Henriques MG. New Therapeutic Targets for the Control of Inflammatory Arthritis: A Pivotal Role for Endothelins, Innovative Rheumatology, Dr. Hiroaki Matsuno (Ed.), InTech. Jan 2013.

[13] Dayer JM. The pivotal role of interleukin-1 in the clinical manifestations of rheumatoid arthritis (in Eng). Rheumatology (Oxford). May 2003;**42**(Suppl 2):ii3–ii10

[14] Kolaczkowska E, Kubes P. Neutrophil recruitment and function in health and inflammation (in Eng). Nature Review Immunology. Mar 2013;**13**(3):159–175

[15] Wipke BT, Allen PM. Essential role of neutrophils in the initiation and progression of a murine model of rheumatoid arthritis (in Eng). Journal of Immunology. Aug 2001;**167**(3):1601–1608

[16] Bombini G, Canetti C, Rocha FA, Cunha FQ. Tumour necrosis factor-alpha mediates neutrophil migration to the knee synovial cavity during immune inflammation (in Eng). European Journal of Pharmacology. Aug 2004;**496**(1-3):197–204

[17] Guerrero AT. Involvement of LTB4 in zymosan-induced joint nociception in mice: Participation of neutrophils and PGE2 (in Eng). Journal of Leukocyte Biology. Jan 2008;**83**(1):122–130

[18] Wright HL, Moots RJ, Edwards SW. The multifactorial role of neutrophils in rheumatoid arthritis (in Eng). Nature Review Rheumatology. Oct 2014; **10**(10):593–601

[19] Kraan MC, de Koster BM, Elferink JG, Post WJ, Breedveld FC, Tak PP. Inhibition of neutrophil migration soon after initiation of treatment with leflunomide or methotrexate in patients with rheumatoid arthritis: Findings in a prospective, randomized, double-blind clinical trial in fifteen patients (in Eng). Arthritis & Rheumatology. Jul 2000;**43**(7):1488–1495

[20] den Broeder AA, Wanten GJ, Oyen WJ, Naber T, van Riel PL, Barrera P. Neutrophil migration and production of reactive oxygen species during treatment with a fully human anti-tumor necrosis factor-alpha monoclonal antibody in patients with rheumatoid arthritis (in Eng). Journal of Rheumatology. Feb 2003;**30**(2):232–237

[21] Ferrandi C. Phosphoinositide 3-kinase gamma inhibition plays a crucial role in early steps of inflammation by blocking neutrophil recruitment (in Eng). Journal of Pharmacology & Experimental Therapy. Sep 2007;**322**(3):923–930

[22] Khanna D. Natural products as a gold mine for arthritis treatment (in Eng). Current Opinion in Pharmacology. Jun 2007;**7**(3):344–351

[23] Singh R, Akhtar N, Haqqi TM. Green tea polyphenol epigallocatechin-3-gallate: Inflammation and arthritis [corrected] (in Eng). Life Science. Jun 2010;**86**(25-26):907–918

[24] Cross A, Bakstad D, Allen JC, Thomas L, Moots RJ, Edwards SW. Neutrophil gene expression in rheumatoid arthritis (in Eng). Pathophysiology. Oct 2005;**12**(3):191–202

[25] Sadik CD, Kim ND, Luster AD. Neutrophils cascading their way to inflammation (in Eng). Trends in Immunology. Oct 2011;**32**(10):452–460

[26] Semerad CL, Liu F, Gregory AD, Stumpf K, Link DC. G-CSF is an essential regulator of neutrophil trafficking from the bone marrow to the blood (in Eng). Immunity. Oct 2002;**17**(4):413–423

[27] Sanz MJ, Kubes P. Neutrophil-active chemokines in in vivo imaging of neutrophil trafficking (in Eng). European Journal of Immunology. Feb 2012;**42**(2):278–283

[28] Chen M. Neutrophil-derived leukotriene B4 is required for inflammatory arthritis (in Eng). Journal of Experimental Medicine. Apr 2006;**203**(4):837–842

[29] Chou RC. Lipid-cytokine-chemokine cascade drives neutrophil recruitment in a murine model of inflammatory arthritis (in Eng). Immunity. Aug 2010;**33**(2):266–278

[30] Sadik CD, Kim ND, Iwakura Y, Luster AD. Neutrophils orchestrate their own recruitment in murine arthritis through C5aR and FcγR signaling (in Eng). Proceedings of the National Academy of Sciences United States of America. Nov 2012;**109**(46):E3177–E3185

[31] Tarrant TK, Patel DD. Chemokines and leukocyte trafficking in rheumatoid arthritis (in Eng). Pathophysiology. Feb 2006;**13**(1):1–14

[32] Cicchetti G, Allen PG, Glogauer M. Chemotactic signaling pathways in neutrophils: From receptor to actin assembly. (in Eng). Critical Reviews in Oral Biology & Medicine. 2002;**13**(3):220–228

[33] Ley K, Laudanna C, Cybulsky MI, Nourshargh S. Getting to the site of inflammation: The leukocyte adhesion cascade updated. (in Eng), Nature Reviews Immunology. Sep 2007;**7**(9):678–89

[34] Stillie R, Farooq SM, Gordon JR, Stadnyk AW. The functional significance behind expressing two IL-8 receptor types on PMN (in Eng). Journal of Leukocyte Biology. Sep 2009;**86**(3):529–543

[35] Futosi K, Fodor S, Mócsai A. Neutrophil cell surface receptors and their intracellular signal transduction pathways (in Eng). International Immunopharmacology. Nov 2013;**17**(3):638–650

[36] Pillinger MH, Abramson SB. The neutrophil in rheumatoid arthritis (in Eng). Rheumatic Disease Clinics of North America. Aug 1995;**21**(3):691–714

[37] Cedergren J, Forslund T, Sundqvist T, Skogh T. Intracellular oxidative activation in synovial fluid neutrophils from patients with rheumatoid arthritis but not from other arthritis patients (in Eng). Journal of Rheumatology. Nov 2007;**34**(11):2162–2170

[38] Hitchon CA, El-Gabalawy HS. Oxidation in rheumatoid arthritis (in Eng). Arthritis Research & Therapy. 2004;**6**(6):265–278

[39] Rasheed Z. Hydroxyl radical damaged immunoglobulin G in patients with rheumatoid arthritis: Biochemical and immunological studies (in Eng). Clinical Biochemistry. Jun 2008;**41**(9):663–669

[40] Elsaid KA, Jay GD, Chichester CO. Detection of collagen type II and proteoglycans in the synovial fluids of patients diagnosed with non-infectious knee joint synovitis indicates early damage to the articular cartilage matrix (in Eng). Osteoarthritis Cartilage. Sep 2003;**11**(9):673–680

[41] Katano M. Implication of granulocyte-macrophage colony-stimulating factor induced neutrophil gelatinase-associated lipocalin in pathogenesis of rheumatoid arthritis revealed by proteome analysis (in Eng). Arthritis & Research Therapy. 2009;**11**(1):R3

[42] Wang CH. Expression of CD147 (EMMPRIN) on neutrophils in rheumatoid arthritis enhances chemotaxis, matrix metalloproteinase production and invasiveness of synoviocytes (in Eng). Journal of Cell & Molecular Medicine. Apr 2011;**15**(4):850–860

[43] Lefrançais E. IL-33 is processed into mature bioactive forms by neutrophil elastase and cathepsin G (in Eng). Proceedings of the National Academy of Sciences United States of America. Jan 2012;**109**(5):1673–1678

[44] Wittkowski H. Effects of intra-articular corticosteroids and anti-TNF therapy on neutrophil activation in rheumatoid arthritis (in Eng). Annals in Rheumatic Diseases. Aug 2007;**66**(8):1020–1025

[45] Conte FP, Menezes-de-Lima O, Verri WA, Cunha FQ, Penido C, Henriques MG. Lipoxin A(4) attenuates zymosan-induced arthritis by modulating endothelin-1 and its effects (in Eng). British Journal of Pharmacology. Oct 2010;**161**(4):911–924

[46] Mathis S, Jala VR, Haribabu B. Role of leukotriene B4 receptors in rheumatoid arthritis (in Eng). Autoimmunity Reviews. Nov 2007;**7**(1):12–17

[47] Firestein, GS. Immunologic Mechanisms in the Pathogenesis of Rheumatoid Arthritis. Journal of Clinical Rheumatology. June 2005; **11**(3):S39–S44

[48] Mantovani A, Cassatella MA, Costantini C, Jaillon S. Neutrophils in the activation and regulation of innate and adaptive immunity (in Eng). Nature Review Immunology. Aug 2011;**11**(8):519–531

[49] Catrina AI, Svensson CI, Malmström V, Schett G, Klareskog L. Mechanisms leading from systemic autoimmunity to joint-specific disease in rheumatoid arthritis (in Eng). Nature Review Rheumatology. Feb 2017;**13**(2):79–86

[50] Khandpur R. NETs are a source of citrullinated autoantigens and stimulate inflammatory responses in rheumatoid arthritis (in Eng). Science Translational Medicine. Mar 2013;**5**(178):178ra40

[51] Cross A, Bucknall RC, Cassatella MA, Edwards SW, Moots RJ. Synovial fluid neutrophils transcribe and express class II major histocompatibility complex molecules in rheumatoid arthritis (in Eng). Arthritis & Rheumatology. Oct 2003;**48**(10):2796–2806

[52] Woodfin A, Voisin MB, Nourshargh S. Recent developments and complexities in neutrophil transmigration (in Eng). Current Opinion in Hematology. Jan 2010;**17**(1):9–17

[53] Chakravarti A, Raquil MA, Tessier P, Poubelle PE. Surface RANKL of Toll-like receptor 4-stimulated human neutrophils activates osteoclastic bone resorption (in Eng). Blood. Aug 2009;**114**(8):1633–1644

[54] Assi LK, et al. Tumor necrosis factor alpha activates release of B lymphocyte stimulator by neutrophils infiltrating the rheumatoid joint (in Eng). Arthritis & Rheumatology. Jun 2007;**56**(6):1776–1786

[55] Cascão R, Rosário HS, Souto-Carneiro MM, Fonseca JE. Neutrophils in rheumatoid arthritis: More than simple final effectors (in Eng). Autoimmunity Review. Jun 2010;**9**(8):531–535

[56] Németh T, Mócsai A. The role of neutrophils in autoimmune diseases (in Eng). Immunology Letters. Mar 2012;**143**(1):9–19

[57] Soehnlein O, Steffens S, Hidalgo A, Weber C. Neutrophils as protagonists and targets in chronic inflammation. Nature Review Immunology, Apr 2017; **17**(4):248–261

[58] Eggleton P, Wang L, Penhallow J, Crawford N, Brown KA. Differences in oxidative response of subpopulations of neutrophils from healthy subjects and patients with rheumatoid arthritis (in Eng). Annals in Rheumatic Diseases. Nov 1995;**54**(11):916–923

[59] Wright HL, Chikura B, Bucknall RC, Moots RJ, Edwards SW. Changes in expression of membrane TNF, NF-{kappa}B activation and neutrophil apoptosis during active and resolved inflammation (in Eng). Annals in Rheumatic Diseases. Mar 2011;**70**(3):537–543

[60] Rollet-Labelle E, Vaillancourt M, Marois L, Newkirk MM, Poubelle PE, Naccache PH. Cross-linking of IgGs bound on circulating neutrophils leads to an activation of endothelial cells: Possible role of rheumatoid factors in rheumatoid arthritis-associated vascular dysfunction (in Eng). Journal of Inflammation (London). Jul 2013;**10**(1):27

[61] Kundu S, Ghosh P, Datta S, Ghosh A, Chattopadhyay S, Chatterjee M. Oxidative stress as a potential biomarker for determining disease activity in patients with rheumatoid arthritis (in Eng). Free Radical Research. Dec 2012;**46**(12);1482–1489

[62] Khojah HM, Ahmed S, Abdel-Rahman MS, Hamza AB. Reactive oxygen and nitrogen species in patients with rheumatoid arthritis as potential biomarkers for disease activity and the role of antioxidants (in Eng). Free Radical Biology Medicine. Aug 2016;**97**:285–291

[63] Murphy G, Nagase H. Reappraising metalloproteinases in rheumatoid arthritis and osteoarthritis: destruction or repair? (in Eng). Nature Clinical Practice Rheumatology. Mar 2008;**4**(3):128–135

[64] Ren K, Dubner R. Interactions between the immune and nervous systems in pain (in Eng). Nature Medicine. Nov 2010;**16**(11):1267–1276

[65] McDougall JJ. Arthritis and pain. Neurogenic origin of joint pain (in Eng). Arthritis & Research Therapy. 2006;**8**(6):220

[66] Schaible HG, Ebersberger A, Von Banchet GS. Mechanisms of pain in arthritis (in Eng). Annals of the New York Academy of Sciences. Jun 2002;**966**:343–354

[67] Schaible HG, Grubb BD. Afferent and spinal mechanisms of joint pain (in Eng). Pain. Oct 1993;**55**(1):5–54

[68] Arend WP, Dayer JM. Inhibition of the production and effects of interleukin-1 and tumor necrosis factor alpha in rheumatoid arthritis (in Eng). Arthritis & Rheumatology. Feb 1995;**38**(2):151–160

[69] Brennan FM, McInnes IB. Evidence that cytokines play a role in rheumatoid arthritis (in Eng). Journal of Clinical Investigation. Nov 2008;**118**(11):3537–3545

[70] Pinto LG, et al. IL-17 mediates articular hypernociception in antigen-induced arthritis in mice (in Eng). Pain. Feb 2010;**148**(2):247–256

[71] Ferreira SH, Romitelli M, de Nucci G. Endothelin-1 participation in overt and inflammatory pain (in Eng). Journal of Cardiovascular Pharmacology. 1989;**13**(Suppl 5):S220–2

[72] Verri WA, Schivo IR, Cunha TM, Liew FY, Ferreira SH, Cunha FQ. Interleukin-18 induces mechanical hypernociception in rats via endothelin acting on ETB receptors in a morphine-sensitive manner (in Eng). Journal of Pharmacology & Experimental Therapy. Aug 2004;**310**(2):710–717

[73] Verri WA, et al. IL-15 mediates immune inflammatory hypernociception by triggering a sequential release of IFN-gamma, endothelin, and prostaglandin (in Eng). Proceedings of the National Academy of Science United States of America. Jun 2006;**103**(25):9721–9725

[74] Verri WA, et al. Antigen-induced inflammatory mechanical hypernociception in mice is mediated by IL-18 (in Eng). Brain Behavioral Immunology. Jul 2007;**21**(5):535–543

[75] Wang ZQ, et al. A newly identified role for superoxide in inflammatory pain (in Eng). Journal of Pharmacology & Experimental Therapy. Jun 2004;**309**(3):869–878

[76] Ting E, et al. Role of complement C5a in mechanical inflammatory hypernociception: potential use of C5a receptor antagonists to control inflammatory pain (in Eng). British Journal of Pharmacology. Mar 2008;**153**(5):1043–1053

[77] Cunha TM, et al. Crucial role of neutrophils in the development of mechanical inflammatory hypernociception (in Eng). Journal of Leukocyte Biology. Apr 2008;**83**(4):824–832

[78] Gokin AP, Fareed MU, Pan HL, Hans G, Strichartz GR, Davar G. Local injection of endothelin-1 produces pain-like behavior and excitation of nociceptors in rats (in Eng). Journal of Neuroscience. Jul 2001;**21**(14):5358–5366

[79] Tanaka D, Kagari T, Doi H, Shimozato T. Essential role of neutrophils in anti-type II collagen antibody and lipopolysaccharide-induced arthritis (in Eng). Immunology. Oct 2006;**119**(2):195–202

[80] Kidd BA, et al. Epitope spreading to citrullinated antigens in mouse models of autoimmune arthritis and demyelination (in Eng). Arthritis & Research Therapy. 2008;**10**(5):R119

[81] Brink M, et al. Anti-carbamylated protein antibodies in the pre-symptomatic phase of rheumatoid arthritis, their relationship with multiple anti-citrulline peptide antibodies and association with radiological damage (in Eng). Arthritis & Research Therapy. Feb 2015;**17**:25

[82] Sokolove J, et al. Autoantibody epitope spreading in the pre-clinical phase predicts progression to rheumatoid arthritis (in Eng). PLoS One. 2012;**7**(5):e35296

[83] van de Stadt LA, et al. Development of the anti-citrullinated protein antibody repertoire prior to the onset of rheumatoid arthritis (in Eng). Arthritis Rheumatology. Nov 2011;**63**(11):3226–3233

[84] Lundberg K, et al. Citrullinated proteins have increased immunogenicity and arthritogenicity and their presence in arthritic joints correlates with disease severity (in Eng). Arthritis & Research Therapy. 2005;**7**(3):R458–67

[85] Sokolove J, Zhao X, Chandra PE, Robinson WH. Immune complexes containing citrullinated fibrinogen costimulate macrophages via Toll-like receptor 4 and Fcγ receptor (in Eng). Arthritis Rheumatology. Jan 2011;**63**(1):53–62

[86] Kinloch A, et al. Identification of citrullinated alpha-enolase as a candidate autoantigen in rheumatoid arthritis (in Eng). Arthritis & Research Therapy. 2005;**7**(6):R1421–9

[87] Cunha TM, Verri WA, Silva JS, Poole S, Cunha FQ, Ferreira SH. A cascade of cytokines mediates mechanical inflammatory hypernociception in mice (in Eng). Proceedings of the National Academy of Sciences United States of America. Feb 2005;**102**(5):1755–1760

[88] Guerrero AT, et al. Toll-like receptor 2/MyD88 signaling mediates zymosan-induced joint hypernociception in mice: Participation of TNF-α, IL-1β and CXCL1/KC (in Eng). European Journal of Pharmacology. Jan 2012;**674**(1):51–57

[89] Qin X, Wan Y, Wang X. CCL2 and CXCL1 trigger calcitonin gene-related peptide release by exciting primary nociceptive neurons (in Eng). Journal of Neuroscience Research. Oct 2005;**82**(1):51–62

[90] Zhang ZJ, Cao DL, Zhang X, Ji RR, Gao YJ. Chemokine contribution to neuropathic pain: respective induction of CXCL1 and CXCR2 in spinal cord astrocytes and neurons (in Eng). Pain. Oct 2013;**154**(10):2185–2197

[91] Matsubara S, Yamamoto T, Tsuruta T, Takagi K, Kambara T. Complement C4-derived monocyte-directed chemotaxis-inhibitory factor. A molecular mechanism to cause polymorphonuclear leukocyte-predominant infiltration in rheumatoid arthritis synovial cavities (in Eng). American Journal of Pathology. May 1991;**138**(5):1279–1291

[92] Papayannopoulos V, Zychlinsky A. NETs: A new strategy for using old weapons (in Eng). Trends in Immunology. Nov 2009;**30**(11):513–521

[93] Brinkmann V, et al. Neutrophil extracellular traps kill bacteria (in Eng). Science. Mar 2004;**303**(5663):1532–1535

[94] Steinberg BE, Grinstein S. Unconventional roles of the NADPH oxidase: signaling, ion homeostasis, and cell death (in Eng). Science STKE. Mar 2007;**2007**(379):pe11

[95] Fuchs TA, et al. Novel cell death program leads to neutrophil extracellular traps (in Eng). Journal of Cell Biology. Jan 2007;**176**(2):231–241

[96] Remijsen Q, Kuijpers TW, Wirawan E, Lippens S, Vandenabeele P, Vanden Berghe T. Dying for a cause: NETosis, mechanisms behind an antimicrobial cell death modality (in Eng). Cell Death Differentiation. Apr 2011;**18**(4):581–588

[97] Wang Y, et al. Histone hypercitrullination mediates chromatin decondensation and neutrophil extracellular trap formation (in Eng). Journal of Cell Biology. Jan 2009;**184**(2): 205–213

[98] Martinod K, et al. Neutrophil histone modification by peptidylarginine deiminase 4 is critical for deep vein thrombosis in mice (in Eng). Proceedings of the National Academy of Sciences United States of America. May 2013;**110**(21):8674–8679

[99] Gupta AK, Giaglis S, Hasler P, Hahn S. Efficient neutrophil extracellular trap induction requires mobilization of both intracellular and extracellular calcium pools and is modulated by cyclosporine A (in Eng). PLoS One. 2014;**9**(5):e97088

[100] Sur Chowdhury C, Giaglis S, Walker UA, Buser A, Hahn S, Hasler P. Enhanced neutrophil extracellular trap generation in rheumatoid arthritis: Analysis of underlying signal transduction pathways and potential diagnostic utility (in Eng). Arthritis & Research Therapy. Jun 2014;**16**(3):R122

[101] Wang Y, et al. Increased neutrophil elastase and proteinase 3 and augmented NETosis are closely associated with β-cell autoimmunity in patients with type 1 diabetes (in Eng). Diabetes. Dec 2014;**63**(12):4239–4248

[102] Kessenbrock K, et al. Netting neutrophils in autoimmune small-vessel vasculitis (in Eng). Nature Medicine. Jun 2009;**15**(6):623–625

[103] Lande R, et al. Neutrophils activate plasmacytoid dendritic cells by releasing self-DNA-peptide complexes in systemic lupus erythematosus (in Eng). Science Translational Medicine. Mar 2011;**3**(73):73ra19

[104] Leffler J, Stojanovich L, Shoenfeld Y, Bogdanovic G, Hesselstrand R, Blom AM. Degradation of neutrophil extracellular traps is decreased in patients with antiphospholipid syndrome (in Eng). Clinical Experimental Rheumatology. Jan-Feb 2014;**32**(1): 66–70

[105] Villanueva E, et al. Netting neutrophils induce endothelial damage, infiltrate tissues, and expose immunostimulatory molecules in systemic lupus erythematosus (in Eng). Journal of Immunology. Jul 2011;**187**(1):538–552

[106] Kaplan MJ, Radic M. Neutrophil extracellular traps: Double-edged swords of innate immunity (in Eng). Journal of Immunology. Sep 2012;**189**(6):2689–2695

[107] Brinkmann V, Zychlinsky A. Neutrophil extracellular traps: Is immunity the second function of chromatin? (in Eng). Journal of Cell Biology. Sep 2012;**198**(5):773–783

[108] Giaglis S, Hahn S, Hasler P. The NET outcome: Are neutrophil extracellular traps of any relevance to the pathophysiology of autoimmune disorders in childhood? (in Eng). Frontiers in Pediatrics. 2016;**4**:97

[109] Sur Chowdhury C, Hahn S, Hasler P, Hoesli I, Lapaire O, Giaglis S. Elevated levels of total cell-free DNA in maternal serum samples arise from the generation of neutrophil extracellular traps (in Eng). Fetal Diagnosis and Therapy. 2016;**40**(4):263–267

[110] Giaglis S, et al. Neutrophil migration into the placenta: Good, bad or deadly? (in Eng). Cell Adhesion and Migration. Mar 2016;**10**(1-2):208–225

[111] Mayadas TN, Cullere X, Lowell CA. The multifaceted functions of neutrophils (in Eng). Annual Review of Pathology. 2014;**9**:181–218

[112] Cross A, Barnes T, Bucknall RC, Edwards SW, Moots RJ. Neutrophil apoptosis in rheumatoid arthritis is regulated by local oxygen tensions within joints (in Eng). Journal of Leukocyte Biology. Sep 2006;**80**(3):521–528

[113] Lally F, et al. A novel mechanism of neutrophil recruitment in a coculture model of the rheumatoid synovium (in Eng). Arthritis & Rheumatology. Nov 2005;**52**(11):3460–3469

[114] Parsonage G, et al. Prolonged, granulocyte-macrophage colony-stimulating factor-dependent, neutrophil survival following rheumatoid synovial fibroblast activation by IL-17 and TNFalpha (in Eng). Arthritis and Research Therapy. 2008;**10**(2):R47

[115] Raza K, et al. Synovial fluid leukocyte apoptosis is inhibited in patients with very early rheumatoid arthritis (in Eng). Arthritis and Research Therapy. 2006;**8**(4):R120

[116] Weinmann P, et al. Delayed neutrophil apoptosis in very early rheumatoid arthritis patients is abrogated by methotrexate therapy (in Eng). Clinical and Experimental Rheumatology. Nov-Dec 2007;**25**(6):885–887

[117] Bendele A. Animal models of rheumatoid arthritis (in Eng). Journal of Musculoskeletal and Neuronal Interactions. Jun 2001;**1**(4):377–385

[118] Asquith DL, Miller AM, McInnes IB, Liew FY. Animal models of rheumatoid arthritis (in Eng). European Journal of Immunology. Aug 2009;**39**(8):2040–2044

[119] Verri WA, et al. IL-33 induces neutrophil migration in rheumatoid arthritis and is a target of anti-TNF therapy (in Eng). Annals in Rheumatic Diseases. Sep 2010;**69**(9):1697–1703

[120] Verri WA, Cunha TM, Parada CA, Poole S, Cunha FQ, Ferreira SH. Hypernociceptive role of cytokines and chemokines: Targets for analgesic drug development? (in Eng). Pharmacological Therapy. Oct 2006;**112**(1):116–138

[121] Smolen JS, Aletaha D, Koeller M, Weisman MH, Emery P. New therapies for treatment of rheumatoid arthritis (in Eng). Lancet. Dec 2007;**370**(9602):1861–1874

[122] Burmester GR, Feist E, Dörner T. Emerging cell and cytokine targets in rheumatoid arthritis (in Eng). Nature Reviews Rheumatology. Feb 2014;**10**(2):77–88

[123] McInnes IB, Liew FY. Cytokine networks—Towards new therapies for rheumatoid arthritis (in Eng). Nature Clinical Practice Rheumatology. Nov 2005;**1**(1):31–39

[124] Wright HL, Moots RJ, Bucknall RC, Edwards SW. Neutrophil function in inflammation and inflammatory diseases (in Eng). Rheumatology (Oxford). Sep 2010;**49**(9):1618–1631

[125] Derouet M, et al. Sodium salicylate promotes neutrophil apoptosis by stimulating caspase-dependent turnover of Mcl-1 (in Eng). Journal of Immunology. Jan 2006;**176**(2): 957–965

[126] Pillinger MH, et al. Modes of action of aspirin-like drugs: Salicylates inhibit ERK activation and integrin-dependent neutrophil adhesion (in Eng). Proceedings of the National Academy of Sciences United States of America. Nov 1998;**95**(24):14540–14545

[127] Neal TM, Vissers MC, Winterbourn CC. Inhibition by nonsteroidal anti-inflammatory drugs of superoxide production and granule enzyme release by polymorphonuclear leukocytes stimulated with immune complexes or formyl-methionyl-leucyl-phenylalanine (in Eng). Biochemical Pharmacology. Aug 1987;**36**(15):2511–2517

[128] Dinarello CA. Anti-inflammatory agents: Present and future (in Eng). Cell. Mar 2010;**140**(6):935–950

[129] Liu L, et al. Rapid non-genomic inhibitory effects of glucocorticoids on human neutrophil degranulation (in Eng). Inflammation Research. Jan 2005;**54**(1):37–41

[130] Crockard AD, Boylan MT, Droogan AG, McMillan SA, Hawkins SA. Methylprednisolone-induced neutrophil leukocytosis—Down-modulation of neutrophil L-selectin and Mac-1 expression and induction of granulocyte-colony stimulating factor (in Eng). International Journal of Clinical and Laboratory Research. 1998;**28**(2):110–115

[131] Youssef PP, et al. Neutrophil trafficking into inflamed joints in patients with rheumatoid arthritis, and the effects of methylprednisolone (in Eng). Arthritis and Rheumatology. Feb 1996;**39**(2):216–225

[132] Majumdar S, Aggarwal BB. Methotrexate suppresses NF-kappaB activation through inhibition of IkappaBalpha phosphorylation and degradation (in Eng). Journal of Immunology. Sep 2001;**167**(5):2911–2920

[133] Sperling RI, Benincaso AI, Anderson RJ, Coblyn JS, Austen KF, Weinblatt ME. Acute and chronic suppression of leukotriene B4 synthesis ex vivo in neutrophils from patients with rheumatoid arthritis beginning treatment with methotrexate (in Eng). Arthritis and Rheumatology. Apr 1992;**35**(4):376–384

[134] Wessels JA, Huizinga TW, Guchelaar HJ. Recent insights in the pharmacological actions of methotrexate in the treatment of rheumatoid arthritis (in Eng). Rheumatology (Oxford). Mar 2008;**47**(3):249–255

[135] Dewas C, Dang PM, Gougerot-Pocidalo MA, El-Benna J. TNF-alpha induces phosphorylation of p47(phox) in human neutrophils: partial phosphorylation of p47phox is a common event of priming of human neutrophils by TNF-alpha and granulocyte-macrophage colony-stimulating factor (in Eng). Journal of Immunology. Oct 2003;**171**(8):4392–4398

[136] Fujishima S, et al. Regulation of neutrophil interleukin 8 gene expression and protein secretion by LPS, TNF-alpha, and IL-1 beta (in Eng). Journal of Cell Physiology. Mar 1993;**154**(3):478–485

[137] Cross A, Moots RJ, Edwards SW. The dual effects of TNFalpha on neutrophil apoptosis are mediated via differential effects on expression of Mcl-1 and Bfl-1 (in Eng). Blood. Jan 2008;**111**(2):878–884

[138] Ginis I, Tauber AI. Activation mechanisms of adherent human neutrophils (in Eng). Blood. Sep 1990;**76**(6):1233–1239

[139] Mitoma H, et al. Mechanisms for cytotoxic effects of anti-tumor necrosis factor agents on transmembrane tumor necrosis factor alpha-expressing cells: comparison among infliximab, etanercept, and adalimumab (in Eng). Arthritis and Rheumatology. May 2008;**58**(5):1248–1257

[140] Taylor PC, et al. Reduction of chemokine levels and leukocyte traffic to joints by tumor necrosis factor alpha blockade in patients with rheumatoid arthritis (in Eng). Arthritis and Rheumatology. Jan 2000;**43**(1):38–47

[141] Dominical VM, et al. Neutrophils of rheumatoid arthritis patients on anti-TNF-α therapy and in disease remission present reduced adhesive functions in association with decreased circulating neutrophil-attractant chemokine levels (in Eng). Scandinavian Journal of Immunology. Apr 2011;**73**(4):309–318

[142] Smolen JS, et al. Effect of interleukin-6 receptor inhibition with tocilizumab in patients with rheumatoid arthritis (OPTION study): A double-blind, placebo-controlled, randomised trial (in Eng). Lancet. Mar 2008;**371**(9617):987–997

[143] Marin V, Montero-Julian F, Grès S, Bongrand P, Farnarier C, Kaplanski G. Chemotactic agents induce IL-6Ralpha shedding from polymorphonuclear cells: Involvement of a metalloproteinase of the TNF-alpha-converting enzyme (TACE) type (in Eng). European Journal of Immunology. Oct 2002;**32**(10):2965–2970

[144] Wright HL, Cross AL, Edwards SW, Moots RJ. Effects of IL-6 and IL-6 blockade on neutrophil function in vitro and in vivo (in Eng). Rheumatology (Oxford). Jul 2014;**53**(7):1321–1331

[145] Yen JH. Treatment of early rheumatoid arthritis in developing countries. Biologics or disease-modifying anti-rheumatic drugs? (in Eng). Biomedicine & Pharmacotherapy. Dec 2006;**60**(10):688–692

[146] Kikuchi M, Matsuura K, Matsumoto Y, Inagaki T, Ueda R. Bibliographical investigation of complementary alternative medicines for osteoarthritis and rheumatoid arthritis (in Eng). Geriatrics & Gerontology International. Mar 2009;**9**(1):29–40

[147] Marcus DM. Therapy: Herbals and supplements for rheumatic diseases (in Eng). Nature Reviews Rheumatology. Jun 2009;**5**(6):299–300

[148] Ernst E. Prevalence of use of complementary/alternative medicine: A systematic review (in Eng). Bulletin of the World Health Organization. 2000;**78**(2):252–257

[149] Steinhubl SR. Why have antioxidants failed in clinical trials? (in Eng). American Journal of Cardiology. May 2008;**101**(10A):14D–19D

[150] Haseeb A, Haqqi TM. Immunopathogenesis of osteoarthritis (in Eng). Clinical Immunology. Mar 2013;**146**(3):185–196

[151] Newman DJ, Cragg GM. Natural products as sources of new drugs over the 30 years from 1981 to 2010 (in Eng). Journal of Natural Products. Mar 2012;**75**(3):311–335

[152] Rothwell JA, et al. Phenol-Explorer 3.0: A major update of the Phenol-Explorer database to incorporate data on the effects of food processing on polyphenol content (in Eng). Database (Oxford). 2013;**2013**:bat070

[153] Kelly GS. Quercetin. Monograph (in Eng). Alternative Medicine Review. Jun 2011;**16**(2):1 72–194

[154] Lamson DW, Brignall MS. Antioxidants and cancer, part 3: Quercetin (in Eng). Alternative Medic ine Review. Jun 2000;**5**(3):196–208

[155] Russo M, Spagnuolo C, Tedesco I, Bilotto S, Russo GL. The flavonoid quercetin in disease prevention and therapy: Facts and fancies (in Eng). Biochemical Pharmacology. Jan 2012;**83**(1):6–15

[156] Gardi C, et al. Quercetin reduced inflammation and increased antioxidant defense in rat adjuvant arthritis (in Eng). Archives of Biochemistry and Biophysics. Oct 2015;**583**:150–157

[157] Pincemail J, Deby C, Thirion A, de Bruyn-Dister M, Goutier R. Human myeloperoxidase activity is inhibited in vitro by quercetin. Comparison with three related compounds (in Eng). Experientia. May 1988;**44**(5):450–453

[158] Suri S, et al. A comparative study of the effects of quercetin and its glucuronide and sulfate metabolites on human neutrophil function in vitro (in Eng). Biochemical Pharmacology. Sep 2008;**76**(5):645–653

[159] Petri B, Phillipson M, Kubes P. The physiology of leukocyte recruitment: An in vivo perspective (in Eng). Journal of Immunology. May 2008;**180**(10):6439–6446

[160] Valério DA, et al. Quercetin reduces inflammatory pain: Inhibition of oxidative stress and cytokine production (in Eng). Journal of Natural Products. Nov 2009;**72**(11):1975–1979

[161] Suyenaga ES, et al. Beyond organoleptic characteristics: The pharmacological potential of flavonoids and their role in leukocyte migration and in L-selectin and β2-integrin expression during inflammation (in Eng). Phytotherapy Research. Sep 2014;**28**(9):1406–1411

[162] Souto FO, et al. Quercetin reduces neutrophil recruitment induced by CXCL8, LTB4, and fMLP: Inhibition of actin polymerization (in Eng). Journal of Natural Products. Feb 2011;**74**(2):113–118

[163] Medeiros KCP, Monteiro JC, Diniz MFFM, Medeiros IA, Silva BA, Piuvezam MR. Effect of the activity of the Brazilian polyherbal formulation: *Eucalyptus globulus* Labill, *Peltodon radicans* Pohl and *Schinus terebinthifolius* Raddi in inflammatory models. Brazilian Journal of Pharmacognosy, Mar 2007; **17**:23–28

[164] Cavalher-Machado SC, et al. The anti-allergic activity of the acetate fraction of Schinus terebinthifolius leaves in IgE induced mice paw edema and pleurisy (in Eng). International Immunopharmacology. Nov 2008;**8**(11):1552–1560

[165] de Lima MR, et al. Anti-bacterial activity of some Brazilian medicinal plants (in Eng). Journal of Ethnopharmacology. Apr 2006;**105**(1-2):137–147

[166] Velázquez E, Tournier HA, Mordujovich de Buschiazzo P, Saavedra G, Schinella GR. Antioxidant activity of Paraguayan plant extracts (in Eng). Fitoterapia. Feb 2003;**74**(1-2):91–97

[167] Rosas EC, et al. Anti-inflammatory effect of Schinus terebinthifolius Raddi hydroalcoholic extract on neutrophil migration in zymosan-induced arthritis (in Eng). Journal of Ethnopharmacology. Dec 2015;**175**:490–498

[168] Whang WK, et al. Methyl gallate and chemicals structurally related to methyl gallate protect human umbilical vein endothelial cells from oxidative stress (in Eng). Experimental & Molecular Medicine. Aug 2005;**37**(4):343–352

[169] Acharyya S, Sarkar P, Saha DR, Patra A, Ramamurthy T, Bag PK. Intracellular and membrane-damaging activities of methyl gallate isolated from *Terminalia chebula* against multidrug-resistant *Shigella* spp. (in Eng). Journal of Medical Microbiology. Aug 2015;**64**(8):901–909

[170] Lee SH, et al. Antitumor activity of methyl gallate by inhibition of focal adhesion formation and Akt phosphorylation in glioma cells (in Eng). Biochimica et Biophysica Acta. Aug 2013;**1830**(8):4017–4029

[171] Correa LB, et al. Anti-inflammatory effect of methyl gallate on experimental arthritis: Inhibition of neutrophil recruitment, production of inflammatory mediators, and activation of macrophages (in Eng). Journal of Natural Products. Jun 2016;**79**(6):1554–1566

[172] Henriques M, Penido C. The therapeutic properties of Carapa guianensis (in Eng). Current Pharmaceutical Design. 2014;**20**(6):850–856

[173] Hammer ML, Johns EA. Tapping an Amazônian plethora: Four medicinal plants of Marajó Island, Pará (Brazil) (in Eng). Journal of Ethnopharmacology. Sep 1993;**40**(1):53–75

[174] Penido C, Conte FP, Chagas MS, Rodrigues CA, Pereira JF, Henriques MG. Anti-inflammatory effects of natural tetranortriterpenoids isolated from *Carapa guianensis* Aublet on zymosan-induced arthritis in mice (in Eng). Inflammation Research. Nov 2006;**55**(11):457–464

[175] Patwardhan CA, Fauq A, Peterson LB, Miller C, Blagg BS, Chadli A. Gedunin inactivates the co-chaperone p23 protein causing cancer cell death by apoptosis (in Eng). Journal of Biological Chemistry. Mar 2013;**288**(10):7313–7325

[176] Conte FP, et al. Effect of gedunin on acute articular inflammation and hypernociception in mice (in Eng). Molecules. 2015;**20**(2):2636–2657

[177] Bozza PT, Bakker-Abreu I, Navarro-Xavier RA, Bandeira-Melo C. Lipid body function in eicosanoid synthesis: An update (in Eng). Prostaglandins, Leukotrienes, & Essential Fatty Acids. Nov 2011;**85**(5):205–213

[178] Khan N, Afaq F, Saleem M, Ahmad N, Mukhtar H. Targeting multiple signaling pathways by green tea polyphenol (-)-epigallocatechin-3-gallate (in Eng). Cancer Research. Mar 2006;**66**(5):2500–2505

[179] Haqqi TM, et al. Prevention of collagen-induced arthritis in mice by a polyphenolic fraction from green tea (in Eng). Proceedings of the National Academy of Sciences United States of America. Apr 1999;**96**(8):4524–4529

[180] Ahmed S, Wang N, Lalonde M, Goldberg VM, Haqqi TM. Green tea polyphenol epigallocatechin-3-gallate (EGCG) differentially inhibits interleukin-1 beta-induced expression of matrix metalloproteinase-1 and -13 in human chondrocytes (in Eng). Journal of Pharmacological & Experimental Therapy. Feb 2004;**308**(2):767–773

[181] Ahmed S, Anuntiyo J, Malemud CJ, Haqqi TM. Biological basis for the use of botanicals in osteoarthritis and rheumatoid arthritis: A review (in Eng). Evidence Based Complementary and Alternative Medicine. Sep 2005;**2**(3):301–308

[182] Ahmed S, et al. Epigallocatechin-3-gallate inhibits IL-6 synthesis and suppresses trans-signaling by enhancing soluble gp130 production (in Eng). Proceedings of the National Academy of Sciences United States of America. Sep 2008;**105**(38):14692–14697

[183] Singh R, Ahmed S, Islam N, Goldberg VM, Haqqi TM. Epigallocatechin-3-gallate inhibits interleukin-1beta-induced expression of nitric oxide synthase and production of nitric oxide in human chondrocytes: Suppression of nuclear factor kappaB activation by degradation of the inhibitor of nuclear factor kappaB (in Eng). Arthritis & Rheumatology. Aug 2002;**46**(8):2079–2086

[184] Yun HJ, Yoo WH, Han MK, Lee YR, Kim JS, Lee SI. Epigallocatechin-3-gallate suppresses TNF-alpha -induced production of MMP-1 and -3 in rheumatoid arthritis synovial fibroblasts (in Eng). Rheumatology International. Nov 2008;**29**(1):23–29

[185] Aktas O, et al. Green tea epigallocatechin-3-gallate mediates T cellular NF-kappa B inhibition and exerts neuroprotection in autoimmune encephalomyelitis (in Eng). Journal of Immunology. Nov 2004;**173**(9):5794–5800

[186] Donà M, et al. Neutrophil restraint by green tea: inhibition of inflammation, associated angiogenesis, and pulmonary fibrosis (in Eng). Journal of Immunology. Apr 2003;**170**(8):4335–4341

[187] Westacott CI, Sharif M. Cytokines in osteoarthritis: Mediators or markers of joint destruction? (in Eng). Seminars in Arthritis & Rheumatology. Feb 1996;**25**(4):254–272

[188] Porath D, Riegger C, Drewe J, Schwager J. Epigallocatechin-3-gallate impairs chemokine production in human colon epithelial cell lines (in Eng). Journal of Pharmacology & Experimental Therapy. Dec 2005;**315**(3):1172–1180

[189] Netsch MI, Gutmann H, Aydogan C, Drewe J. Green tea extract induces interleukin-8 (IL-8) mRNA and protein expression but specifically inhibits IL-8 secretion in caco-2 cells (in Eng). Planta Medica. Jun 2006;**72**(8):697–702

[190] Park C, et al. Curcumin induces apoptosis and inhibits prostaglandin E(2) production in synovial fibroblasts of patients with rheumatoid arthritis (in Eng). International Journal of Molecular Medicine. Sep 2007;**20**(3):365–372

[191] Mun SH, et al. Oral administration of curcumin suppresses production of matrix metalloproteinase (MMP)-1 and MMP-3 to ameliorate collagen-induced arthritis: Inhibition of the PKCdelta/JNK/c-Jun pathway (in Eng). Journal of Pharmacological Science. Sep 2009;**111**(1):13–21

[192] Kloesch B, Becker T, Dietersdorfer E, Kiener H, Steiner G. Anti-inflammatory and apoptotic effects of the polyphenol curcumin on human fibroblast-like synoviocytes (in Eng). International Immunopharmacology. Feb 2013;**15**(2):400–405

[193] Kim DC, Lee W, Bae JS. Vascular anti-inflammatory effects of curcumin on HMGB1-mediated responses in vitro (in Eng). Inflammation Research. Dec 2011;**60**(12):1161–1168

[194] Chandran B, Goel A. A randomized, pilot study to assess the efficacy and safety of curcumin in patients with active rheumatoid arthritis (in Eng). Phytotherapy Research. Nov 2012;**26**(11):1719–1725

[195] Di Pierro F, Rapacioli G, Di Maio EA, Appendino G, Franceschi F, Togni S. Comparative evaluation of the pain-relieving properties of a lecithinized formulation of curcumin (Meriva(®)), nimesulide, and acetaminophen (in Eng). Journal of Pain Research. 2013;**6**:201–205

[196] Belcaro G, et al. Efficacy and safety of Meriva®, a curcumin-phosphatidylcholine complex, during extended administration in osteoarthritis patients (in Eng). Alternative Medicine Review. Dec 2010;**15**(4):337–344

Chapter 6

Role of Neutrophils in Cystic Fibrosis Lung Disease

Massimo Conese, Stefano Castellani,
Susanna D'Oria, Sante Di Gioia and
Pasqualina Montemurro

Additional information is available at the end of the chapter

http://dx.doi.org/10.5772/67798

Abstract

Cystic fibrosis (CF) is a genetic syndrome caused by mutations in the *CF Transmembrane Conductance Regulator (CFTR)* gene. In CF patients, chief morbidity and mortality are due to pulmonary manifestations. CFTR lack/dysfunction brings an altered ion flux through the airway epithelium and ablation of mucociliary clearance, which in turn ensues in colonization and infection by opportunistic bacterial pathogens and subsequent neutrophil-dominated inflammation. This response eventually leads to the damage of the lung tissue. A host of inflammatory mediators attract, activate, and reprogramme neutrophils to survive (avoiding apoptosis) and produce a wealth of proteases and radical oxygen species. The protease/antiprotease imbalance and oxidative stress have multiple downstream effects, including impaired mucus clearance, increased and self-perpetuating inflammation, and impaired immune responses, thus facilitating and fostering bacterial infections. On the other hand, CFTR lack or dysfunction is likely responsible for alterations in neutrophils concerning chemotaxis, phagocytosis, oxidative burst, degranulation, and neutrophil extracellular trap (NET) formation. A good opportunity to reveal new and non-invasive biomarkers of CF lung disease is the evaluation of circulating neutrophils. Indeed, neutrophil responses are now investigated as outcomes of the aetiological therapies in CF, such as hypertonic saline, antiproteases, CFTR correctors and potentiators.

Keywords: neutrophils, cystic fibrosis, proteases, NETs, oxidative burst, degranulation, chemotaxis

1. Introduction

Cystic fibrosis (CF) is a rare autosomal recessive disease whose average birth incidence rate is now 2.9/10,000 (i.e. 1/3500) in Europe [1] and prevalence is 100,000 globally [2]. Although CF is a chronic disease affecting many organs, the lung manifestations are still today the major cause of morbidity and mortality of these individuals and are the consequences of an ongoing inflammatory process, which stems either in the absence or in the presence of opportunistic bacterial infections. Lung inflammation and respiratory infections affect the prognosis of CF patients [3, 4]; indeed, they are associated with the progressive destructive changes that are responsible for most of the morbidity and mortality in CF [5]. Over 1000 microbial species (viruses, bacteria, mould, and fungi) have been found in the airways of CF patients [6]. *Staphylococcus aureus* and *Haemophilus influenzae* are the most common pathogens isolated from the sputum in the first decade of life, while *Pseudomonas aeruginosa* is found to dominate numerically in the second and third decades of life [7]. However, according to the Cystic Fibrosis Foundation Registry, *P. aeruginosa* is no longer the most common pathogen cultured in individuals with CF in the USA, and there has been an increase in the prevalence of *S. aureus* and *Stenotrophomonas maltophilia* [8].

Mutations in the 250-kb *CF transmembrane conductance regulator (CFTR)* gene are responsible for CF, but other environmental and genetic modifiers are thought to play a role in the phenotype of lung disease [9]. The CFTR gene encodes for a chloride channel that is expressed on the apical membrane of epithelial cells residing in organs with absorptive/secretory properties (**Figure 1(a)**). More than 2000 mutations have been identified at the moment (www.genet.sickkids.on.ca/cftr/), which can be classified in six classes (**Table 1**).

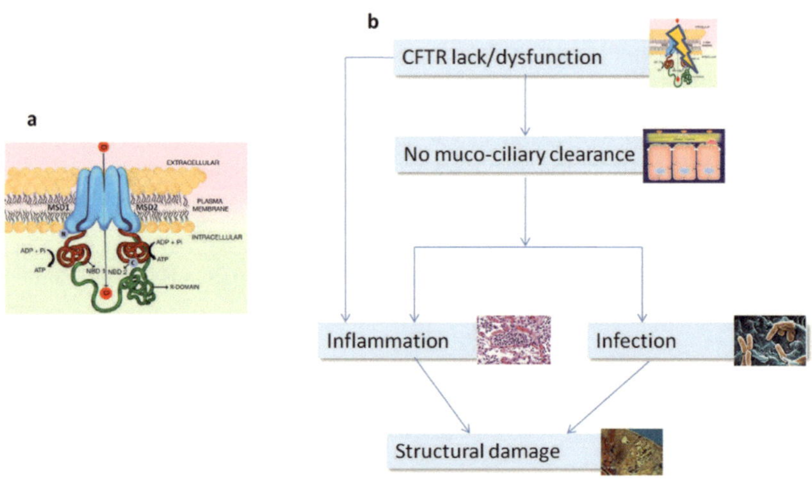

Figure 1. CFTR structure and CF lung disease. (a) A supposed CFTR structure when inserted in the plasma membrane. CFTR is composed of a two-membrane spanning domain (MSDs), each linked to nucleotide-binding domains (NBD1 and NBD2). Unique to CFTR, NBD1 is connected to the NBD2 by a regulatory domain (R). (b) The pathophysiological cascade of CF lung disease.

CFTR mutation class	Example	Effect on CFTR protein
Class I (stop mutation)	G542X	No expression
Class II (trafficking mutants)	F508del	Very low expression
Class III (low ATP binding)	G551D	Very low function
Class IV (low conductance)	R117H	Low function
Class V (low synthesis)	A455E	Low expression
Class VI (high turnover)	120del23	Low expression

Table 1. The six classes of CFTR mutations and their effects at the protein level.

The hallmark of the CF lung disease is a neutrophil-dominated inflammatory response; however, the link between CFTR mutations and the complex inflammatory milieu of the CF lungs is largely still poorly understood. The pathophysiological cascade which leads from the lack/dysfunction of CFTR chloride channel activity to the airway inflammation and infection, and eventually to tissue damage and destruction, is represented in **Figure 1(c)**. In the airways, the low excretion of chloride ions and bicarbonate, along with the hyperabsorption of sodium by the epithelial sodium channel (ENaC) and subsequently of water, contributes to the volume depletion from the periciliary liquid and its acidification. Thus, the loss of CFTR reduces the effectiveness of at least two defences—mucociliary transport and antimicrobial activity [10–12]. This eventually brings the colonization and infection by opportunistic bacterial pathogens and opposing inflammation, which, far from being resolutive, seems to be dysregulated, becoming chronic. In this context, polymorphonuclear leukocytes (PMNs) are thought to play a fundamental role on the onset and progression of lung tissue damage. Observational clinical studies made in the past have ascertained that infants with CF do show an airway inflammation prior to overt infection [13], indicating that the inflammatory response is dysregulated a priori before any bacterial infection and also suggesting that CFTR mutations are implicated in this abnormal response (**Figure 1(b)**). This is supported by the findings showing that free and bound airway neutrophil elastase is detected very early in CF infants and predicts the development of bronchiectasis later in life [14]. Furthermore, it has been found that CFTR is involved in some functions of innate immune cells that are diverted by CFTR mutations. We will discuss these evidences in Section 4.

2. Recruitment and activation of neutrophils in CF lungs

Neutrophils are the main cell types involved in the first-line defence of many organs, including the respiratory tract. However, they remain in the blood circulation unless they are recruited in the tissue. In the airways, they are marginated along the endothelium of capillaries and are ready to migrate first through the endothelium and then across the respiratory epithelium [15]. Marginated neutrophils are recruited rapidly to sites of inflammation, where their primary role is to kill invading bacteria and certain fungal species through phagocytosis and production of a range of oxygen species within the phagolysosomes and also by preformed granular enzymes and proteins. Tissue inflammation results in the release of multiple inflammatory mediators and subsequent neutrophil priming. Priming results in a marked change in neutrophil shape and rheology that leads to their increased stiffness and retention within the capillary microvascular bed of the lung [16]. These mediators include an early wave comprised of cytokines, such as tumour necrosis factor (TNF)-α, interleukin (IL)-1β, and pathogen-associated molecular patterns (PAMPs) such as endotoxin, the ligand of Toll-like receptor (TLR)-4, followed by a late wave of chemoattractants and growth factors including IL-8, leukotriene B_4 (LTB_4), and granulocyte-macrophage colony-stimulating factor (GM-CSF).

In the airways, macrophages and epithelial cells are the main cell types which sense the pathogens and secrete a wealth of factors both inducing priming and full activation of neutrophils, as well as their extravasation. Upon exposure to bacteria, respiratory epithelial cells release reactive oxygen species (ROS) as an innate anti-infective mechanism, together with several anti-microbial peptides such as human beta-defensins (hBD-1/2/4) and cathelicidins (LL-37). The major pro-inflammatory cytokines (e.g. IL-1β, TNF-α, and IL-6) are initially expressed and released by surface epithelial cells of the conductive airways, which also release chemokines directed to recruit neutrophils (e.g. IL-8, GRO-α/γ) [17–22]. Besides the phagocytosis of inhaled pathogens and apoptotic cells, alveolar macrophages (AMs) play an important role in orchestrating innate immune defences by releasing inflammatory mediators. One of the important regulatory functions of AMs may be to dampen immune responses [23] so that dysfunction of AMs in CF could be related to increased inflammation. Both airway epithelial cells and AMs have been shown to be dysfunctional in CF, contributing to the onset and progression of chronic lung disease [24, 25]. This is reflected by the high burden of cytokines, chemokines, and other mediators found in the airway secretion of CF patients [26]. The CF airways contain massive amounts of cytokines and chemoattractants for neutrophils such as TNF-α, IL-1β, IL-6, IL-8, IL-17, IL-33, LTB_4, C5a, high-mobility group box 1 (HMGB1), proline-glycine-proline (PGP), and N-acetyl PGP [27–32]. For example, TNF-α enhances the neutrophil oxidative capacity, the granule release, and, with IL-1β, induces the priming of neutrophils [33]. The concentration of IL-8 in bronchoalveolar lavage (BAL) fluid is generally elevated and often correlates with the number of neutrophils in the airways [34]. It is thought that both extrinsic (e.g. microbes) and intrinsic (e.g. *CFTR* mutations) contribute to the alterations of the respiratory epithelium and AMs, ensuing in a hyper-inflammatory state and defect in immune defence.

Besides chemokines, such as CXCL8 (IL-8) [35], and lipid products, such as LTB_4 [36], other mediators have also been recently implicated in the recruitment of neutrophils into the CF airways. UDP-glucose levels are abnormally elevated in lung secretions from CF patients and from a mouse model of CF/chronic bronchitis, the βENaC-Tg transgenic mouse [37]. Moreover, instillation of UDP-glucose into mouse lung resulted in robust accumulation of neutrophils in BAL. Levels of damage-associated molecular patterns (DAMP), HMGB1, were found elevated in CF sputum and in BAL from βENaC-Tg transgenic mouse and shown to be chemotactic for neutrophils [38]. Upon activation, neutrophils secrete matrix metalloproteinases (MMP)-8 and -9, which perform an initial digestion of collagen from the macromolecule's size. Subsequently, neutrophils release prolyl endopeptidase (PE), a serine protease

http://dx.doi.org/10.5772/67798

previously only known to be a processor of neuropeptides. PE performs the final digestion of collagen to the tri-peptide PGP, which, upon binding to the same receptors as IL-8, CXCR1 and CXCR2, acts as a neutrophil chemoattractant and activator [39]. Thus, release of this peptidic collagen fragment provides a positive feedback mechanism that contributes to persistent neutrophilic inflammation in the CF lung [40]. During the adaptive immune response phase, neutrophils are recruited to the lung via the IL-23/IL-17A axis. Dendritic cells, activated by bacterial antigens, produce IL-23, which, in turn, binds to IL-23 receptor on T cells and stimulates them to produce IL-17A. This cytokine induces granulopoiesis via the induction of G-CSF and neutrophil recruitment via induction of chemotactic mediators such as IL-8. Both IL-23 and IL-17A have been found at high levels in the sputum from CF patients in acute exacerbation [41] and in stable condition [42], amplifying the extravasation and activation of neutrophils already induced by the innate immune response.

Once extravasated, neutrophils locate all along the CF bronchial tree and particularly in segmental bronchi, where they preferentially locate at the level of the lamina propria and in the lumen [43]. In this position, they are already activated and try to phagocytose microbes (e.g. *P. aeruginosa*) which have adapted to the hypoxic environment by producing an exopolysaccharide called alginate [44]. This frustrated phagocytosis leads to neutrophil hyperactivation which is more harmful than protective.

In the following subsections, we shall revise the main features of neutrophil physiology and how these are modified in the CF airway microenvironment (**Figure 2**).

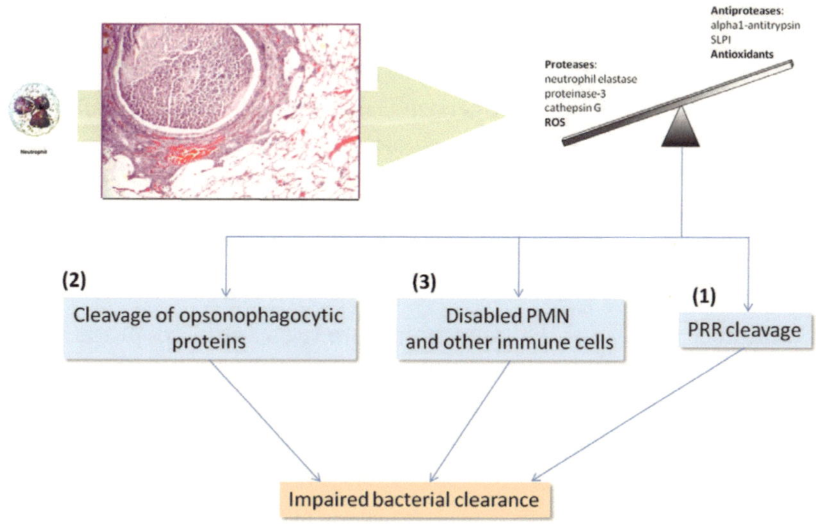

Figure 2. The role of neutrophils in maintaining inflammation and respiratory infections. The increased burden of neutrophils in the CF airways is the hallmark of the mucus plugs contained in the bronchioles lumen. From this location, PMNs secrete proteases and reactive oxygen species that overwhelm antiproteases and antioxidants, respectively, ensuing in various effects: (1) cleavage of pattern recognition receptors (PRR), (2) cleavage of opsonophagocytic receptors, and (3) disabling PMNs themselves and other immune cells. All these alterations facilitate bacterial infections.

2.1. Activation

Neutrophils recruited from the blood into the CF airway environment undergo marked functional changes. They express high levels of markers conventionally found on long-lived antigen-presenting cells (APCs), including class II molecules of the Major Histocompatibility Complex (MHC), the costimulatory molecule CD80, and the chemoattractant receptor of Th2 cells (CD294), all of which suggest profound reprogramming [45]. CF airway neutrophils present marked increases in glucose, amino acid, and phosphate transporters as compared with blood neutrophils [46], indicating that metabolic adaptation of neutrophils occurs as they are recruited to CF airways. However, these changes are not equal for all neutrophil subsets found in CF airways.

2.2. Apoptosis and resolution of inflammation

Apoptosis is a physiological process necessary for the clearance of inflammatory cells. Neutrophils are short-living cells which undergo apoptosis at the end of the inflammatory response, attracting macrophages which eventually ingest apoptotic cells in a process called *efferocytosis*. The removal of apoptotic cells is relevant to avoid secondary necrosis and the release of pro-inflammatory mediators that disrupt tissue homeostasis [47]. In CF, the lung disease is characterized by an altered balance of pro- and anti-inflammatory mediators. Studies have shown that CF airways are deficient in several anti-inflammatory molecules, including IL-10 and lipoxin-A_4 (LXA_4) [48]. IL-10 inhibits the pro-inflammatory activities of cytokines, chemokines, and transcription factors and induces neutrophil apoptosis [49]. Not surprisingly, IL-10 knockout mice inoculated with *P. aeruginosa* that was embedded in agarose beads, in order to mimic a chronic Pseudomonas infection, had more drastic weight loss, greater neutrophil infiltration, larger inflammatory exudate of the lungs, and higher concentrations of pro-inflammatory cytokines in BAL compared to wild-type mice [50, 51]. Lipoxins are arachidonic metabolites generated by a lipoxigenase transcellular pathway involving neutrophils with epithelia, endothelia, monocytes, and platelets. In particular, LXA_4 acts to down-modulate acute inflammation by inhibiting neutrophil transmigration induced by LTB_4 and IL-8 and stimulating macrophage phagocytosis of apoptotic PMNs [52, 53]. LXA_4 levels have been found to be reduced in BAL fluid from CF patients, along with a significant suppression of LXA_4/neutrophil ratios [54, 55].

It seems for a number of reasons that neutrophils are resistant to apoptosis when they have extravasated into the CF airways; for example, it has been suggested that the oversecretion of cytokines might be responsible of apoptosis inhibition of airway neutrophils. The release of G-CSF or GM-CSF by epithelial cells, stimulated by *S. aureus* or *P. aeruginosa*, inhibits apoptosis of CF neutrophils [56], suggesting that increased expression of cytokines by CF airway cells not only induces neutrophil response but also enhances their survival, perpetuating an inflammatory process. Also, it has been described that PMNs from CF patients showed delayed constitutive and TNF-α or GM-CSF-induced phosphatidylinositol 3-kinase (PI3K)-dependent apoptosis [57]. CF airway neutrophils also undergo strong activation of CREB and mTOR's pro-survival pathways [58]. Moreover, it has been postulated that delayed phosphatidylserine externalization and mitochondria depolarization might be responsible for delayed apoptosis of CF neutrophils [59]. In another study [60], neutrophils isolated from CF patients showed enhanced survival and upregulation of p21/Waf1, a cyclin-dependent kinase inhibitor and partner of proliferating cell nuclear antigen (PCNA). As also suggested by in vivo studies in p21(−/−) mice with *P. aeruginosa* lipopolysaccharide (LPS) challenge, p21/Waf1 is involved in the apoptotic response occurring during the resolution of inflammation [60]. In order to dissect the early phases of interaction between CF neutrophils and airway epithelial cells, it was found in co-culture experiments that a high number of non-apoptotic airway PMNs adhered to the CF airway epithelium in the presence of elevated levels of IL-6 and IL-8 [61], indicating another mechanism involved in enhanced inflammatory responses in airways of CF patients. Finally, independent of the sensitivity to apoptosis of CF cells, it has been shown that clearance of apoptotic cells by efferocytosis is defective in CF due to elastase-mediated degradation of macrophage phosphatidylserine receptors and that accumulation of such cells may contribute to ongoing inflammation [62].

2.3. Phagocytosis, oxidative burst, and degranulation

In cystic fibrosis, there is a tendency for bacterial colonization that may be due to dysfunction of phagocytosis. Airway neutrophils of CF patients showed a blunted phagocytic capacity and a reduced expression of cell surface recognition receptors, namely TLRs, leading to impaired bacterial killing [63]. Recent studies have demonstrated that CF neutrophils display an absence or dysfunction of CFTR at the level of phagolysosomes [64]. Likely due to this defect, CF neutrophils are impaired in chlorination of engulfed pathogens due to defective hypochlorous acid (HOCl) production [65].

One of the major mechanisms through which neutrophil phagocytosis kills pathogens entrapped inside the phagolysosomal vacuole is the release of high quantities of ROS [66]. The activation of the nicotinamide adenine dinucleotide phosphate oxidase (NOX2) in the neutrophils induces the production of superoxide anion and consequently the other ROS. Excessive activation of the neutrophil NOX2 results in exaggerated ROS release in the external surroundings, which increases the oxidative damage to tissues [67]. Furthermore, the inflammatory response can be enhanced by imbalance created by excessive release of pro-oxidative and impaired release of anti-oxidative molecules. While some authors have reported that ROS production by CF blood PMNs can be higher than or identical to that of healthy controls [68, 69], others have demonstrated that ROS generation varied according to the infecting pathogen [70] or to the method employed to detect respiratory burst activity [71]. For example, it has been shown that an extracellular polysaccharide of non-mucoid *P. aeruginosa* strain (Psl) inhibits opsonization and reduces ROS production by neutrophils [72]. Montemurro et al. [73] have established that CF blood neutrophils at the baseline are characterized by a higher ROS release as compared with controls PMNs and that the antibiotic therapy does not change this pattern. Nevertheless, ROS production is reduced in airway neutrophils compared to blood neutrophils that have different ROS oxidant activity profiles [74].

Neutrophils are identified by the presence of cytoplasmic primary (azurophilic), secondary (specific), and tertiary (gelatinase) granules as well as the secretory vesicles [75]. Focusing on granules, neutrophils abundantly express a cell-type specific set of neutrophil serine proteases, namely cathepsin G, proteinase 3, and neutrophil elastase (NE), which are stored in the azurophilic granules. Also, myeloperoxidase (MPO) is stored in primary granules. Secondary granules are characterized by the presence of lactoferrin and cathelicidins, such as hCAP-18, while tertiary granules are enriched with gelatinase, an old name for MMPs, in particular MMP-9.

A dysregulated neutrophil degranulation capacity in CF has been shown. Neutrophils obtained from CF patients have an increased capacity to release primary granule contents such as MPO and NE [76]. In the airways, CF neutrophils undergo active exocytosis of primary granules, leading to a massive release of enzymes (e.g. NE, MPO) that damage the airway tissue and perpetuate inflammation [45]. On the other hand, Pohl et al. [77] have demonstrated that blood neutrophils obtained from CF patients can release less secondary (lactoferrin and hCAP-18) and tertiary (MMP-9) granule components compared with cells obtained from healthy individuals. The dysfunction of CFTR channel in neutrophils results in the deactivation of the GTP-binding protein Rab27a and in an impaired granule exocytosis. Interestingly, hypoxia, which is a hallmark of the CF bronchiolar environment, augmented neutrophil degranulation and possibly enhanced damage to respiratory airway cells in a hypoxia-inducible factor (HIF)-independent but PI3Kγ-dependent mechanism [78].

2.4. NETosis

The neutrophils are the first immune cells to achieve the site of injury or infection and are key players in microbial killing, because they are equipped with three main anti-bacterial weapons: phagocytosis, release of ROS, and granule release. Aside from these traditional mechanisms, neutrophils are also able, upon activation, to release DNA fibres decorated with anti-microbial proteins or neutrophil extracellular traps (NETs) to immobilize and to kill bacteria. NETs are composed of chromatin fibres coated with anti-microbial proteins, such as histones, NE, MPO, and α-defensins [79–82]. Moreover, NETs and their associated molecules are able to directly induce epithelial death, and massive NET formation has been reported in several pulmonary diseases including CF [83]. NETs are present in excess in CF sputum and the normal host defence functions become pathological [84]. CF patients with poor pulmonary functions presented higher levels of NETs compared to patients with mild lung disease, and the G protein-coupled receptor (GPCR) CXCR2 mediates NOX2-independent NET formation [85]. Histones and protease-coated DNA structures are released by neutrophils in response to respiratory bacteria (whole cells or virulence factors such as LPS, pilus, pyocyanin) or to inflammatory mediators (IL-8, interferon type I [IFN I], C5a) [86]. The exotoxin pyocyanin, a virulence factor of *P. aeruginosa,* enhances NET formation and requires NOX2 for its action [87]. Another pro-inflammatory cytokine, macrophage migration inhibitory factor (MIF), is able to stimulate NET release by promoting mitogen-activated protein kinase and thus exacerbating the inflammation [88]. Finally, *P. aeruginosa* triggers the release by lung epithelial cells of the eicosanoid hepoxilin A3, a neutrophil chemoattractant that induces NETosis [89]. Besides, MPO and NE expressed on NET fibres may induce the degradation of proteins of the connective tissue and of endothelial heparan sulphate proteoglycan at the site of inflammation [90, 91], contributing to lung pathology of CF patients. Furthermore, there is growing evidence of NET escape by pathogens. NET release might be inhibited by down-regulation of inflammatory responses, or NET degradation might be induced by bacteria, including *H. influenzae*, by deoxyribonuclease [92]. Also *P. aeruginosa*, a very mutable bacterium, is able to acquire resistance to NET-mediated killing [93].

2.5. Cytokine production and immune regulation

As already pointed out above, there are many synergistic mediators which prime, activate, and attract neutrophils in the CF airways. Neutrophils also contribute to the CF airway environment by producing mediators that are pro-inflammatory and modify the function of other immune cells. CF airway neutrophils were found to increase TLR-4 expression on their surface and produce excessive IL-8 at the baseline, while failing to increase secretion in response to LPS or repress it in response to IL-10 [94]. Neutrophils in the sputum and blood of F508del CF subjects at the time of pulmonary exacerbation were found to express IL-17 RNA and protein as well as IL-23 receptor [95]. These investigators also showed a positive correlation between percent-IL-17-producing neutrophils and the total sputum activity of NE and MMP-9 and that IL-17 was absent following antibiotic treatment. IL-17 production by neutrophils may therefore contribute to tissue damage in the lungs of patients with CF.

Neutrophilic myeloid-derived suppressor cells (MDSC) are innate immune cells that are functionally characterized by their potential to suppress T- and natural killer (NK)-cell responses. Circulating neutrophilic MDSC have been found to be increased in patients with CF infected with *P. aeruginosa* as compared with age-matched healthy control subjects, their percentages correlating with lung function in those patients [96]. Further studies have revealed in an in vivo animal model of respiratory infection that *P. aeruginosa* triggers the recruitment of neutrophilic MDSC into the pulmonary compartment and enhances their suppressive capacity towards T cells [97]. Interestingly, they also showed that MDSC obtained from Cftr$^{-/-}$ mice were generated and recruited as in wild-type mice but were impaired in suppressing T-cell proliferation compared to their *Cftr*$^{+/+}$ counterpart cells. Thus, neutrophils contribute to the escape of *P. aeruginosa* from the adaptive immune response, and *CFTR* mutations may contribute to the bacterial infection.

3. Neutrophils and the effect of *CFTR* mutations

While bacteria and their products, cytokines and chemokines, are important triggers of neutrophil activation in CF airways, it is an emerging picture that a primary CFTR defect in cells of the innate immune system, including neutrophils, monocytes, and lymphocytes, contributes significantly to CF lung pathology [24]. Pharmacologic inhibition of CFTR and genetic mutation (F508del) in murine neutrophils activated the nuclear factor kappa-light-chain enhancer of activated B cells (NF-κB) and increased macrophage inflammatory protein-2 (MIP-2) and TNF-α production, as compared to non-inhibited and control neutrophils. Interestingly, under LPS challenge, neutrophil-depleted wild-type mice reconstituted with F508del neutrophils displayed a more severe lung inflammation in comparison with neutrophil-depleted wild-type mice reconstituted with wild-type neutrophils [98]. Altogether, these data strongly indicate that the lack of functional CFTR could result in excessive NF-κB activation in neutrophils and therefore propagate a hyper-inflammatory response.

CF neutrophils have a reduced phagocytic activity [19, 99] and defects in the respiratory burst, attributed to disrupted chloride transport to the phagolysosome [65, 100–102]. While wild-type CFTR is transported to neutrophil phagosomes, the F508del protein is not targeted efficiently to these organelles [64], explaining why a correct chlorination of phagosomes in CF does not occur and hence the bactericidal defect. A still debated question is, however, the CFTR expression in neutrophils. Morris and colleagues, although found a defect in iC3b-mediated phagocytosis, did not detect CFTR in circulating and airway neutrophils by either immuno-labelling or a Western blot [99]. Others found that CFTR expression was limited or undetectable in neutrophils by flow cytometry and also that no role for CFTR in neutrophil-mediated phagocytosis was observed [103]. On the other hand, Zhou and colleagues found CFTR at the phagosome level, although a lentiviral-expressing system was used to achieve high protein levels. It might be that CFTR, expressed in hematopoietic stem/progenitor cells [104, 105], is down-regulated to low levels during neutrophil maturation, which is nevertheless sufficient for neutrophil phagocytic and killing activities. The lack/dysfunction of CFTR in the bone marrow may lead to an irreversible functional defect. In this context, it is worth mentioning that knocking out CFTR in the myeloid compartment of mice resulted in poor survival, increased inflammation with recruitment of neutrophils, elevated cytokine production, and inability to resolve infection upon challenge with *P. aeruginosa*-loaded agarose beads to mimic a chronic pulmonary infection [106].

4. Disabling neutrophils and other immune cells in CF airways

Excess neutrophil recruitment to the lungs results in the discharge of their destructive weapons not only directed to kill pathogens (see Section 2) but also to damage the lung and airway tissue. A large number of mediators produced by neutrophils, mainly oxidants and proteases, escape from neutrophils during cell death and phagocytosis. NE, a serine protease capable of digesting several substrates including structural proteins, is a direct mediator degrading elastin, which drives towards bronchiectasis and bronchomalacia [18]. Importantly, NE is associated with lung function decline [107]. In the lung, the main protease inhibitors, the prototypical α1-antitrypsin (α1-AT) secreted by hepatocytes and secretory leukoprotease inhibitor (SLPI) produced by the respiratory epithelium in bronchi and bronchioles, are designed to oppose free proteases and prevent their deleterious effects. These protease inhibitors are eventually overwhelmed by the protease burden in the lung and degraded by bacterial and human NE. It has been documented that despite normal antigenic concentrations of α1-AT and SLPI in children with CF, the majority of α1-AT and SLPI were complexed and/or degraded [108]. In addition, CF airways are exposed to ROS (O_2, H_2O_2, HOCl), derived mainly from the host's immune response. This oxidative stress exacerbates pulmonary deterioration and advances bronchiectasis in patients with CF [109]. Similar to the protease/antiprotease balance, antioxidants produced by airway epithelial cells (reduced glutathione [GSH] and thiocyanate [SCN^-]) are overwhelmed by the burden of oxidants in the CF airways. Activated neutrophils are also capable of oxidizing glutathione by HOCl [110], contributing to GSH deficiency in CF airways. Hypochlorous acid is also able to oxidize calprotectin thereby inhibiting its ability to sequester manganese and zinc ions and consequently to limiting the growth of *S. aureus* and *P. aeruginosa* [111]. Moreover, it has been documented that ROS suppresses CFTR function [112] and that NE degrades CFTR [113], further worsening the CF pathophysiologic vicious cycle.

An important role in the degradation of structural proteins in CF airways is played synergistically by serine proteases, such as NE, proteinase 3, and cathepsin G [114]. In cystic fibrosis, neutrophil activation and degranulation result in the excessive release of proteinase 3, cathepsin G, and NE into the extracellular medium as active enzymes. Part of these serine proteases are exposed at the cell surface of immune cells and are important as modulators of the inflammatory response. Proteinase 3 has been shown to convert IL-8 to more potent, amino-terminally truncated forms [115], indicating that neutrophil proteases released in the inflamed lung convert IL-8 to enhance its chemotactic activity. Besides serine proteases, neutrophil-derived metalloproteinases, including MMP-8 and MMP-9, have also been involved in CF lung disease and chronic neutrophilic inflammation [116]. NE contributes to MMP-9 activation early in CF disease as the ratio of active/pro-enzyme MMP-9 was found to be higher in the presence of free neutrophil elastase activity, but not infection, and active MMP-9 was associated with progression of bronchiectasis [117]. In the context of CF, it is important to recall that neutrophil proteases increase mucin secretion in the airways and reduce ciliary beat frequency, contributing to the impairment in mucociliary clearance [118, 119], induce airway epithelial cells to produce neutrophil chemoattractants [120], and activate the apical epithelial sodium channel ENaC [121].

Unopposed serine proteases and metalloproteinases are responsible for degradation of soluble pattern recognition receptors (PRRs). NE proteolytic activity present in the CF sputum has been shown to degrade the prototypic long pentraxin PTX3, explaining the low levels of this PRR in CF airway secretions [122]. Released cathepsin G upon neutrophil activation degrades both components of the extracellular matrix and the surfactant protein A, a peptide that facilitates bacterial clearance by alveolar macrophages [123]. MMP-9 cleaves the pulmonary collectin surfactant protein D (SP-D) more efficiently than NE; this cleavage causes SP-D to no longer be able to agglutinate bacteria and affects SP-D's innate immune functions, as bacteria are no longer efficiently phagocytosed by alveolar macrophages in vitro [124].

High levels of neutrophil proteases further worsen the immune response by disabling immune cell functions. NE has several potential roles in disabling neutrophils including cleavage of opsonophagocytosis proteins, such as iC3b, complement receptor 1 (CR1) and C5a receptor [125–127], the chemokine receptor CXR1 [128], and TIM3 receptor leading to decreased galectin-9/TIM3 interactions [129]. Overall, the loss of these proteins is responsible for suboptimal local neutrophil priming and bacterial clearance. PMN-derived cathepsin G also thwarts efficient phagocytosis by macrophages, resulting in the cleavage of receptors and causing inefficient opsonization and impaired bacterial killing [18]. Cathepsin G cleavage of serum amyloid P component (SAP) renders it anti-opsonic, as evidenced by the increased binding of SAP to *P. aeruginosa* LPS and inhibition of phagocytosis in vitro [130], thus sequestering bacteria within the lung and potentially contributing to persistent infections in CF. Cathepsin G also interferes with removal of neutrophilic apoptotic bodies, since it mediates the degradation of the macrophage phosphatidylserine receptors with failure to resolve inflammation because of the lack of efferocytosis [62, 131]. Also, NK cells and lymphocytes are disabled by neutrophil serine proteases. Cathepsin G determines a proteolytic cleavage of NKp46, a crucial activating receptor expressed on NK cells, an effect also determined by the CF sputum [132]. NE cleaves T-cell receptors CD2, CD4, CD8, and CD14, impairing monocyte activation and also blocking dendritic cell maturation and antigen presentation [133, 134].

5. Neutrophils as biomarkers of CF lung disease

The mainstays of CF lung disease management are commenced early in infancy and presently include chest physiotherapy to remove mucus plugs from the airways and antibiotic therapy to control infections [12]. Other therapeutic approaches such as hypertonic saline, finalized to increase mucociliary clearance, should be corroborated by efficacy data [135]. Recombinant human DNAse (Dornase alpha) is a strong mucolytic which improves lung function [136] but is given to CF infants only on indication due to its cost [137]. The recent breakthrough in CF, represented by the use of CFTR-correcting therapies, is a milestone in the clinical management of these patients. Ivacaftor (Kalydeco®, Vertex Pharmaceuticals, USA) is a CFTR potentiator given successfully to patients with class III gating mutations. This drug not only improves lung function and normalizes sweat chloride in children above 6 years of age [138], but its efficacy has also been proven in preschoolers [139].

At whatever age, the control of therapeutic efficacy of medications is granted by functional respiratory tests. However, more specific and sensitive assays are urgently needed to monitor the halt in the progression of lung disease, especially now that we entered the era of personalized medicine in CF [140]. Neutrophils, the main cell type involved in the onset and progression of CF lung disease, are clearly an interesting target in this context and are being evaluated for such a purpose. The best indication that neutrophils and their products are sensitive biomarkers of CF lung disease comes from the clinical data about NE. Sputum NE levels have been validated as the most predictive biomarker of lung decline and reduced survival [107, 141], being, however, of no utility in non-expectorating young children. Being easy to isolate from the peripheral blood, circulating neutrophils are more at hand to being studied. Conese et al. [142] analysed blood neutrophils by microarray gene expression in 10 CF patients, homozygous for the F508del mutation, given a course of parenteral antibiotics for an acute exacerbation, before and after therapy. mRNAs of three genes were found downregulated in CF patients before therapy and returned to 'healthy' levels after therapy: phorbol-12-myristate-13-acetate-induced protein 1 (*PMAIP1*), hydrogen voltage-gated channel 1 (*HVCN1*), and β-arrestin 1 (*ARRB1*). Recently, we validated neutrophil *HVCN1* mRNA as a biomarker following the treatment of seven CF patients, homozygous or heterozygous for class III mutations, with ivacaftor, confirming that its expression levels are lower as compared with healthy controls before therapy, while they are increased after CF patients were treated for 6 months (Guerra et al., submitted). Overall, these data strongly indicate that *HVCN1* mRNA level is a neutrophil biomarker sensitive to therapy. In another study [77], ivacaftor treatment resulted in normalized ion homeostasis and corrected Rab27a activation as well as degranulation in blood neutrophils

http://dx.doi.org/10.5772/67798

obtained from six CF patients with the genotype *F508del/G551D*. In line with these findings, extracellular Pseudomonas killing by CF neutrophils obtained from CF patients during treatment was significantly increased. Activated CD11b was investigated as a marker of neutrophil activation and whether it was downregulated by ivacaftor treatment in five patients with *F508del/G551D* and *G551D/N1303K* genotypes [143]. A cytofluorimetric assay showed that activated CD11b on PMNs was significantly higher at baseline in the CF patients compared to controls. However, after treatment, this marker was not significantly different from healthy controls, suggesting that ivacaftor treatment results in a decrease, towards normalization, of the activation status of blood neutrophils in vivo.

6. Conclusion

CF neutrophils display a number of abnormalities including increased survival, hyperactivation with increased protease and ROS production, defects in phagocytosis, and increased NET formation. Altogether, these neutrophil anomalies are derived from an intrinsic CFTR defect and are compounded by bacterial products. The unbalanced protease/antiprotease ratio in favour of proteases is responsible, together with excess oxidative stress, for the structural damage of CF airways and for secondary defects in an innate immune response as well as a skewed adaptive immune response. The neutrophil protease production is thus one of the main targets for therapy today to be explored. CF neutrophils can be also envisaged as a biomarker of therapies. The sensitivity to therapy of neutrophil genes is worthy of further investigation in the clinical setting. A higher number of patients are needed for studies aimed to consider neutrophils and their products as predictors of acute exacerbation and follow up.

Acknowledgements

This work was supported by the Italian Ministry of Health (Law 548/93). Stefano Castellani is a researcher funded by Intervento Cofinanziato dal Fondo di Sviluppo e Coesione 2007–2013—APQ Ricerca Regione Puglia 'Programma regionale a sostegno della specializzazione intelligente e delle sostenibilità sociale ed ambientali—Future In Research'.

Author details

Massimo Conese[1]*, Stefano Castellani[1], Susanna D'Oria[2], Sante Di Gioia[1] and Pasqualina Montemurro[2]

*Address all correspondence to: massimo.conese@unifg.it

1 Department of Medical and Surgical Sciences, University of Foggia, Foggia, Italy

2 Section of General Pathology, Department of Biomedical Sciences and Human Oncology, University of Bari, Bari, Italy

References

[1] Scotet V, Dugueperoux I, Saliou P, Rault G, Roussey M, et al. Evidence for decline in the incidence of cystic fibrosis: a 35-year observational study in Brittany, France. Orphanet J Rare Dis. 2012; **7**: 14.

[2] Davies JC, Ebdon AM, Orchard C. Recent advances in the management of cystic fibrosis. Arch Dis Child. 2014; **99**: 1033–6.

[3] Dakin CJ, Numa AH, Wang H, Morton JR, Vertzyas CC, et al. Inflammation, infection, and pulmonary function in infants and young children with cystic fibrosis. Am J Respir Crit Care Med. 2002; **165**: 904–10.

[4] Pereira LC, Moreira EA, Bennemann GD, Moreno YM, Buss Zda S, et al. Influence of inflammatory response, infection, and pulmonary function in cystic fibrosis. Life Sci. 2014; **109**: 30–6.

[5] Pillarisetti N, Williamson E, Linnane B, Skoric B, Robertson CF, et al. Infection, inflammation, and lung function decline in infants with cystic fibrosis. Am J Respir Crit Care Med. 2011; **184**: 75–81.

[6] Bhagirath AY, Li Y, Somayajula D, Dadashi M, Badr S, et al. Cystic fibrosis lung environment and *Pseudomonas aeruginosa* infection. BMC Pulm Med. 2016; **16**: 174.

[7] Coutinho HD, Falcao-Silva VS, Goncalves GF. Pulmonary bacterial pathogens in cystic fibrosis patients and antibiotic therapy: a tool for the health workers. Int Arch Med. 2008; **1**: 24.

[8] Cystic Fibrosis Foundation. Patient registry 2015 annual report. Bethesda, MD: Cystic Fibrosis Foundation; 2015.

[9] Cutting GR. Cystic fibrosis genetics: from molecular understanding to clinical application. Nat Rev Genet. 2015; **16**: 45–56.

[10] Boucher RC. Airway surface dehydration in cystic fibrosis: pathogenesis and therapy. Annu Rev Med. 2007; **58**: 157–70.

[11] Stoltz DA, Meyerholz DK, Welsh MJ. Origins of cystic fibrosis lung disease. N Engl J Med. 2015; **372**: 351–62.

[12] Proesmans M. Best practices in the treatment of early cystic fibrosis lung disease. Ther Adv Respir Dis. 2017; **11**: 97–104.

[13] Armstrong DS, Grimwood K, Carlin JB, Carzino R, Gutièrrez JP, et al. Lower airway inflammation in infants and young children with cystic fibrosis. Am J Respir Crit Care Med. 1997; **156**: 1197–204.

[14] Sly PD, Gangell CL, Chen L, Ware RS, Ranganathan S, et al. Risk factors for bronchiectasis in children with cystic fibrosis. N Engl J Med. 2013; **368**: 1963–70.

[15] Downey DG, Bell SC, Elborn JS. Neutrophils in cystic fibrosis. Thorax. 2009; **64**: 81–8.

[16] Summers C, Rankin SM, Condliffe AM, Singh N, Peters AM, et al. Neutrophil kinetics in health and disease. Trends Immunol. 2010; **31**: 318–24.

[17] Conese M, Copreni E, Di Gioia S, De Rinaldis P, Fumarulo R. Neutrophil recruitment and airway epithelial cell involvement in chronic cystic fibrosis lung disease. J Cyst Fibros. 2003; **2**: 129–35.

[18] Cohen TS, Prince A. Cystic fibrosis: a mucosal immunodeficiency syndrome. Nat Med. 2012; **18**: 509–19.

[19] Cohen-Cymberknoh M, Kerem E, Ferkol T, Elizur A. Airway inflammation in cystic fibrosis: molecular mechanisms and clinical implications. Thorax. 2013; **68**: 1157–62.

[20] Bezzerri V. Proinflammatory signal transduction in epithelial cells: the model of cystic fibrosis lung disease. Ph.D. thesis, University of Verona, Verona, 2012.

[21] Jacquot J, Tabary O, Le Rouzic P, Clement A. Airway epithelial cell inflammatory signalling in cystic fibrosis. Int J Biochem Cell Biol. 2008; **40**: 1703–15.

[22] Holtzman MJ, Byers DE, Alexander-Brett J, Wang X. The role of airway epithelial cells and innate immune cells in chronic respiratory disease. Nat Rev Immunol. 2014; **14**: 686–98.

[23] Takabayshi K, Corr M, Hayashi T, Redecke V, Beck L, et al. Induction of a homeostatic circuit in lung tissue by microbial compounds. Immunity. 2006; **24**: 475–87.

[24] Ratner D, Mueller C. Immune responses in cystic fibrosis: are they intrinsically defective? Am J Respir Cell Mol Biol. 2012; **46**: 715–22.

[25] Xu Y, Worgall S. Immune dysfunction in cystic fibrosis. In: Sriramulu D, editor. Cystic fibrosis—renewed hopes through research. Rijeka: InTech; 2012, pp. 273–88.

[26] Sagel SD, Chmiel JF, Konstan MW. Sputum biomarkers of inflammation in cystic fibrosis lung disease. Proc Am Thorac Soc. 2007; **4**: 406–17.

[27] Elizur A, Cannon CL, Ferkol TW. Airway inflammation in cystic fibrosis. Chest. 2008; **133**: 489–95.

[28] Dhooghe B, Noel S, Huaux F, Leal T. Lung inflammation in cystic fibrosis: pathogenesis and novel therapies. Clin Biochem. 2014; **47**: 539–46.

[29] Di Gioia S, Sardo C, Castellani S, Porsio B, Belgiovine G, et al. From genesis to revelation: the role of inflammatory mediators in chronic respiratory diseases and their control by nucleic acid-based drugs. Curr Drug Deliv. 2017; 14: 234–52.

[30] Roussel L, Farias R, Rousseau S. IL-33 is expressed in epithelia from patients with cystic fibrosis and potentiates neutrophil recruitment. J Allergy Clin Immunol. 2013; **131**: 913–6.

[31] Sass LA, Hair PS, Perkins AM, Shah TA, Krishna NK, et al. Complement effectors of inflammation in cystic fibrosis lung fluid correlate with clinical measures of disease. PLoS One. 2015; **10**: e0144723.

[32] Gaggar A, Jackson PL, Noerager BD, O'Reilly PJ, McQuaid DB, et al. A novel proteolytic cascade generates an extracellular matrix-derived chemoattractant in chronic neutrophilic inflammation. J Immunol. 2008; **180**: 5662–9.

[33] Hostoffer RW, Krukovets I, Berger M. Enhancement by tumor necrosis factor-alpha of Fc alpha receptor expression and IgA-mediated superoxide generation and killing of Pseudomonas *aeruginosa* by polymorphonuclear leukocytes. J Infect Dis. 1994; **170**: 82–7.

[34] Khan TZ, Wagener JS, Bost T, Martinez J, Accurso FJ, et al. Early pulmonary inflammation in infants with cystic fibrosis. Am J Respir Crit Care Med. 1995; **151**: 1075–82.

[35] Bodas M, Vij N. The NF-kappaB signaling in cystic fibrosis lung disease: pathophysiology and therapeutic potential. Discov Med. 2010 **9**: 346–56.

[36] Ringholz FC, Buchanan PJ, Clarke DT, Millar RG, McDermott M, et al. Reduced 15-lipoxygenase 2 and lipoxin A4/leukotriene B4 ratio in children with cystic fibrosis. Eur Respir J. 2014; **44**: 394–404.

[37] Sesma JI, Weitzer CD, Livraghi-Butrico A, Dang H, Donaldson S, et al. UDP-glucose promotes neutrophil recruitment in the lung. Purinergic Signal. 2016; **12**: 627–35.

[38] Rowe SM, Jackson PL, Liu G, Hardison M, Livraghi A, et al. Potential role of high-mobility group box 1 in cystic fibrosis airway disease. Am J Respir Crit Care Med. 2008; **178**: 822–31.

[39] Guess TA, Gaggar A, Hardison MT. New frontiers in the diagnosis and treatment of chronic neutrophilic lung diseases. In: Kayembe J-M, editor. Oncogenesis, inflammatory and parasitic tropical diseases of the lung. Rijeka: InTech; 2013, pp. 1–24.

[40] Gaggar A, Rowe SM, Matthew H, Blalock JE. Proline-glycine-proline (PGP) and high mobility group box protein-1 (HMGB1): potential mediators of cystic fibrosis airway inflammation. Open Respir Med J. 2010; **4**: 32–8.

[41] McAllister F, Henry A, Kreindler JL, Dubin PJ, Ulrich L, et al. Role of IL-17A, IL-17F, and the IL-17 receptor in regulating growth-related oncogene-alpha and granulocyte colony-stimulating factor in bronchial epithelium: implications for airway inflammation in cystic fibrosis. J Immunol. 2005; **175**: 404–12.

[42] Decraene A, Willems-Widyastuti A, Kasran A, De Boeck K, Bullens DM, et al. Elevated expression of both mRNA and protein levels of IL-17A in sputum of stable cystic fibrosis patients. Respir Res. 2010; **11**: 177.

[43] Hubeau C, Lorenzato M, Couetil JP, Hubert D, Dusser D, et al. Quantitative analysis of inflammatory cells infiltrating the cystic fibrosis airway mucosa. Clin Exp Immunol. 2001; **124**: 69–76.

[44] Cantin AM, Hartl D, Konstan MW, Chmiel JF. Inflammation in cystic fibrosis lung disease: pathogenesis and therapy. J Cyst Fibros. 2015; **14**: 419–30.

[45] Tirouvanziam R, Gernez Y, Conrad CK, Moss RB, Schrijver I, et al. Profound functional and signaling changes in viable inflammatory neutrophils homing to cystic fibrosis airways. Proc Natl Acad Sci USA. 2008; **105**: 4335–9.

[46] Laval J, Touhami J, Herzenberg LA, Conrad C, Taylor N, et al. Metabolic adaptation of neutrophils in cystic fibrosis airways involves distinct shifts in nutrient transporter expression. J Immunol. 2013; **190**: 6043–50.

[47] McCubbrey AL, Curtis JL. Efferocytosis and lung disease. Chest. 2013; **143**: 1750–7.

[48] Bonfield TL, Konstan MW, Berger M. Altered respiratory epithelial cell cytokine production in cystic fibrosis. J Allergy Clin Immunol. 1999; **104**: 72–8.

[49] Cox G. IL-10 enhances resolution of pulmonary inflammation in vivo by promoting apoptosis of neutrophils. Am J Physiol. 1996; **271**: L566–71.

[50] Chmiel JF, Konstan MW, Knesebeck JE, Hilliard JB, Bonfield TL, et al. IL-10 attenuates excessive inflammation in chronic Pseudomonas infection in mice. Am J Respir Crit Care Med. 1999; **160**: 2040–7.

[51] Chmiel JF, Konstan MW, Saadane A, Krenicky JE, Lester Kirchner H, et al. Prolonged inflammatory response to acute Pseudomonas challenge in interleukin-10 knockout mice. Am J Respir Crit Care Med. 2002; **165**: 1176–81.

[52] Karp CL, Flick LM, Yang R, Uddin J, Petasis NA. Cystic fibrosis and lipoxins. Prostaglandins Leukot Essent Fatty Acids. 2005; **73**: 263–70.

[53] Higgins G, Ringholz F, Buchanan P, McNally P, Urbach V. Physiological impact of abnormal lipoxin A(4) production on cystic fibrosis airway epithelium and therapeutic potential. Biomed Res Int. 2015; **2015**: 781087.

[54] Karp CL, Flick LM, Park KW, Softic S, Greer TM, et al. Defective lipoxin-mediated anti-inflammatory activity in the cystic fibrosis airway. Nat Immunol. 2004; **5**: 388–92.

[55] Starosta V, Ratjen F, Rietschel E, Paul K, Griese M. Anti-inflammatory cytokines in cystic fibrosis lung disease. Eur Respir J. 2006; **28**: 581–7.

[56] Saba S, Soong G, Greenberg S, Prince A. Bacterial stimulation of epithelial G-CSF and GM-CSF expression promotes PMN survival in CF airways. Am J Respir Cell Mol Biol. 2002; **27**: 561–7.

[57] McKeon DJ, Condliffe AM, Cowburn AS, Cadwallader KC, Farahi N, et al. Prolonged survival of neutrophils from patients with Delta F508 CFTR mutations. Thorax. 2008; **63**: 660–1.

[58] Makam M, Diaz D, Laval J, Gernez Y, Conrad CK, et al. Activation of critical, host-induced, metabolic and stress pathways marks neutrophil entry into cystic fibrosis lungs. Proc Natl Acad Sci USA. 2009; **106**: 5779–83.

[59] Moriceau S, Kantari C, Mocek J, Davezac N, Gabillet J, et al. Coronin-1 is associated with neutrophil survival and is cleaved during apoptosis: potential implication in neutrophils from cystic fibrosis patients. J Immunol. 2009; **182**: 7254–63.

[60] Martin C, Ohayon D, Alkan M, Mocek J, Pederzoli-Ribeil M, et al. Neutrophil-expressed p21/waf1 favors inflammation resolution in *Pseudomonas aeruginosa* infection. Am J Respir Cell Mol Biol. 2016; **54**: 740–50.

[61] Tabary O, Corvol H, Boncoeur E, Chadelat K, Fitting C, et al. Adherence of airway neutrophils and inflammatory response are increased in CF airway epithelial cell-neutrophil interactions. Am J Physiol Lung Cell Mol Physiol. 2006; **290**: L588–96.

[62] Vandivier RW, Fadok VA, Hoffmann PR, Bratton DL, Penvari C, et al. Elastase-mediated phosphatidylserine receptor cleavage impairs apoptotic cell clearance in cystic fibrosis and bronchiectasis. J Clin Invest. 2002; **109**: 661–70.

[63] Donnelly LE, Barnes PJ. Defective phagocytosis in airways disease. Chest. 2012; **141**: 1055–62.

[64] Zhou Y, Song K, Painter RG, Aiken M, Reiser J, et al. Cystic fibrosis transmembrane conductance regulator recruitment to phagosomes in neutrophils. J Innate Immun. 2013; **5**: 219–30.

[65] Painter RG, Valentine VG, Lanson NA, Jr., Leidal K, Zhang Q, et al. CFTR Expression in human neutrophils and the phagolysosomal chlorination defect in cystic fibrosis. Biochemistry. 2006; **45**: 10260–9.

[66] Amulic B, Cazalet C, Hayes GL, Metzler KD, Zychlinsky A. Neutrophil function: from mechanisms to disease. Annu Rev Immunol. 2012; **30**: 459–89.

[67] El-Benna J, Hurtado-Nedelec M, Marzaioli V, Marie JC, Gougerot-Pocidalo MA, et al. Priming of the neutrophil respiratory burst: role in host defense and inflammation. Immunol Rev. 2016; **273**: 180–93.

[68] Vaisman N, Kerasin E, Hahn T, Trifon S, Voet H, et al. Increased neutrophil chemiluminescence production in patients with cystic fibrosis. Metabolism. 1994; **43**: 719–22.

[69] McKeon DJ, Cadwallader KA, Idris S, Cowburn AS, Pasteur MC, et al. Cystic fibrosis neutrophils have normal intrinsic reactive oxygen species generation. Eur Respir J. 2010; **35**: 1264–72.

[70] Fruhwirth M, Ruedl C, Ellemunter H, Bock G, Wolf H. Flow-cytometric evaluation of oxidative burst in phagocytic cells of children with cystic fibrosis. Int Arch Allergy Immunol. 1998; **117**: 270–5.

[71] Witko-Sarsat V, Allen RC, Paulais M, Nguyen AT, Bessou G, et al. Disturbed myeloperoxidase-dependent activity of neutrophils in cystic fibrosis homozygotes and heterozygotes, and its correction by amiloride. J Immunol. 1996; **157**: 2728–35.

[72] Mishra M, Byrd MS, Sergeant S, Azad AK, Parsek MR, et al. *Pseudomonas aeruginosa* Psl polysaccharide reduces neutrophil phagocytosis and the oxidative response by limiting complement-mediated opsonization. Cell Microbiol. 2012; **14**: 95–106.

[73] Montemurro P, Mariggio MA, Barbuti G, Cassano A, Vincenti A, et al. Increase in interleukin-8 production from circulating neutrophils upon antibiotic therapy in cystic fibrosis patients. J Cyst Fibros. 2012; **11**: 518–24.

[74] Houston N, Stewart N, Smith DS, Bell SC, Champion AC, et al. Sputum neutrophils in cystic fibrosis patients display a reduced respiratory burst. J Cyst Fibros. 2013; **12**: 352–62.

[75] Pham CT. Neutrophil serine proteases: specific regulators of inflammation. Nat Rev Immunol. 2006; **6**: 541–50.

[76] Koller DY, Urbanek R, Gotz M. Increased degranulation of eosinophil and neutrophil granulocytes in cystic fibrosis. Am J Respir Crit Care Med. 1995; **152**: 629–33.

[77] Pohl K, Hayes E, Keenan J, Henry M, Meleady P, et al. A neutrophil intrinsic impairment affecting Rab27a and degranulation in cystic fibrosis is corrected by CFTR potentiator therapy. Blood. 2014; **124**: 999–1009.

[78] Hoenderdos K, Lodge KM, Hirst RA, Chen C, Palazzo SG, et al. Hypoxia upregulates neutrophil degranulation and potential for tissue injury. Thorax. 2016; **71**: 1030–8.

[79] Brinkmann V, Reichard U, Goosmann C, Fauler B, Uhlemann Y, et al. Neutrophil extracellular traps kill bacteria. Science. 2004; **303**: 1532–5.

[80] Urban CF, Reichard U, Brinkmann V, Zychlinsky A. Neutrophil extracellular traps capture and kill *Candida albicans* yeast and hyphal forms. Cell Microbiol. 2006; **8**: 668–76.

[81] McCormick A, Heesemann L, Wagener J, Marcos V, Hartl D, et al. NETs formed by human neutrophils inhibit growth of the pathogenic mold *Aspergillus fumigatus*. Microbes Infect. 2010; **12**: 928–36.

[82] Jenne CN, Wong CH, Zemp FJ, McDonald B, Rahman MM, et al. Neutrophils recruited to sites of infection protect from virus challenge by releasing neutrophil extracellular traps. Cell Host Microbe. 2013; **13**: 169–80.

[83] Saffarzadeh M, Juenemann C, Queisser MA, Lochnit G, Barreto G, et al. Neutrophil extracellular traps directly induce epithelial and endothelial cell death: a predominant role of histones. PLoS One. 2012; **7**: e32366.

[84] Yoo DG, Floyd M, Winn M, Moskowitz SM, Rada B. NET formation induced by *Pseudomonas aeruginosa* cystic fibrosis isolates measured as release of myeloperoxidase-DNA and neutrophil elastase-DNA complexes. Immunol Lett. 2014; **160**: 186–94.

[85] Marcos V, Zhou Z, Yildirim AO, Bohla A, Hector A, et al. CXCR2 mediates NADPH oxidase-independent neutrophil extracellular trap formation in cystic fibrosis airway inflammation. Nat Med. 2010; **16**: 1018–23.

[86] Wartha F, Beiter K, Normark S, Henriques-Normark B. Neutrophil extracellular traps: casting the NET over pathogenesis. Curr Opin Microbiol. 2007; **10**: 52–6.

[87] Rada B, Jendrysik MA, Pang L, Hayes CP, Yoo DG, et al. Pyocyanin-enhanced neutrophil extracellular trap formation requires the NADPH oxidase. PLoS One. 2013; **8**: e54205.

[88] Dwyer M, Shan Q, D'Ortona S, Maurer R, Mitchell R, et al. Cystic fibrosis sputum DNA has NETosis characteristics and neutrophil extracellular trap release is regulated by macrophage migration-inhibitory factor. J Innate Immun. 2014; **6**: 765–79.

[89] Douda DN, Grasemann H, Pace-Asciak C, Palaniyar N. A lipid mediator hepoxilin A3 is a natural inducer of neutrophil extracellular traps in human neutrophils. Mediators Inflamm. 2015; **2015**: 520871.

[90] Logters T, Margraf S, Altrichter J, Cinatl J, Mitzner S, et al. The clinical value of neutrophil extracellular traps. Med Microbiol Immunol. 2009; **198**: 211–9.

[91] Fujie K, Shinguh Y, Inamura N, Yasumitsu R, Okamoto M, et al. Release of neutrophil elastase and its role in tissue injury in acute inflammation: effect of the elastase inhibitor, FR134043. Eur J Pharmacol. 1999; **374**: 117–25.

[92] Storisteanu DM, Pocock JM, Cowburn AS, Juss JK, Nadesalingam A, et al. Evasion of neutrophil extracellular traps by respiratory pathogens. Am J Respir Cell Mol Biol. 2016 Nov 17. [Epub ahead of print].

[93] Young RL, Malcolm KC, Kret JE, Caceres SM, Poch KR, et al. Neutrophil extracellular trap (NET)-mediated killing of *Pseudomonas aeruginosa*: evidence of acquired resistance within the CF airway, independent of CFTR. PLoS One. 2011; **6**: e23637.

[94] Petit-Bertron AF, Tabary O, Corvol H, Jacquot J, Clement A, et al. Circulating and airway neutrophils in cystic fibrosis display different TLR expression and responsiveness to interleukin-10. Cytokine. 2008; **41**: 54–60.

[95] Taylor PR, Bonfield TL, Chmiel JF, Pearlman E. Neutrophils from F508del cystic fibrosis patients produce IL-17A and express IL-23-dependent IL-17RC. Clin Immunol. 2016; **170**: 53–60.

[96] Rieber N, Brand A, Hector A, Graepler-Mainka U, Ost M, et al. Flagellin induces myeloid-derived suppressor cells: implications for *Pseudomonas aeruginosa* infection in cystic fibrosis lung disease. J Immunol. 2013; **190**: 1276–84.

[97] Oz HH, Zhou B, Voss P, Carevic M, Schroth C, et al. *Pseudomonas aeruginosa* airway infection recruits and modulates neutrophilic myeloid-derived suppressor cells. Front Cell Infect Microbiol. 2016; **6**: 167.

[98] Su X, Looney MR, Su HE, Lee JW, Song Y, et al. Role of CFTR expressed by neutrophils in modulating acute lung inflammation and injury in mice. Inflamm Res. 2011; **60**: 619–32.

[99] Morris MR, Doull IJ, Dewitt S, Hallett MB. Reduced iC3b-mediated phagocytotic capacity of pulmonary neutrophils in cystic fibrosis. Clin Exp Immunol. 2005; **142**: 68–75.

[100] Painter RG, Bonvillain RW, Valentine VG, Lombard GA, LaPlace SG, et al. The role of chloride anion and CFTR in killing of *Pseudomonas aeruginosa* by normal and CF neutrophils. J Leukoc Biol. 2008; **83**: 1345–53.

[101] Painter RG, Marrero L, Lombard GA, Valentine VG, Nauseef WM, et al. CFTR-mediated halide transport in phagosomes of human neutrophils. J Leukoc Biol. 2010; **87**: 933–42.

[102] Bonvillain RW, Painter RG, Adams DE, Viswanathan A, Lanson NA, Jr., et al. RNA interference against CFTR affects HL60-derived neutrophil microbicidal function. Free Radic Biol Med. 2010; **49**: 1872–80.

[103] Van de Weert-van Leeuwen PB, Van Meegen MA, Speirs JJ, Pals DJ, Rooijakkers SH, et al. Optimal complement-mediated phagocytosis of *Pseudomonas aeruginosa* by monocytes is cystic fibrosis transmembrane conductance regulator-dependent. Am J Respir Cell Mol Biol. 2013; **49**: 463–70.

[104] Piro D, Rejman J, Conese M. Stem cell therapy for cystic fibrosis: current status and future prospects. Expert Rev Respir Med. 2008; **2**: 365–80.

[105] Trotta T, Guerra L, Piro D, d'Apolito M, Piccoli C, et al. Stimulation of beta2-adrenergic receptor increases CFTR function and decreases ATP levels in murine hematopoietic stem/progenitor cells. J Cyst Fibros. 2015; **14**: 26–33.

[106] Bonfield TL, Hodges CA, Cotton CU, Drumm ML. Absence of the cystic fibrosis transmembrane regulator (Cftr) from myeloid-derived cells slows resolution of inflammation and infection. J Leukoc Biol. 2012; **92**: 1111–22.

[107] Sagel SD, Wagner BD, Anthony MM, Emmett P, Zemanick ET. Sputum biomarkers of inflammation and lung function decline in children with cystic fibrosis. Am J Respir Crit Care Med. 2012; **186**: 857–65.

[108] Birrer P, McElvaney NG, Rudeberg A, Sommer CW, Liechti-Gallati S, et al. Protease-antiprotease imbalance in the lungs of children with cystic fibrosis. Am J Respir Crit Care Med. 1994; **150**: 207–13.

[109] Galli F, Battistoni A, Gambari R, Pompella A, Bragonzi A, et al. Oxidative stress and antioxidant therapy in cystic fibrosis. Biochim Biophys Acta. 2012; **1822**: 690–713.

[110] Kettle AJ, Turner R, Gangell CL, Harwood DT, Khalilova IS, et al. Oxidation contributes to low glutathione in the airways of children with cystic fibrosis. Eur Respir J. 2014; **44**: 122–9.

[111] Magon NJ, Turner R, Gearry RB, Hampton MB, Sly PD, et al. Oxidation of calprotectin by hypochlorous acid prevents chelation of essential metal ions and allows bacterial growth: relevance to infections in cystic fibrosis. Free Radic Biol Med. 2015; **86**: 133–44.

[112] Cantin AM, Bilodeau G, Ouellet C, Liao J, Hanrahan JW. Oxidant stress suppresses CFTR expression. Am J Physiol Cell Physiol. 2006; **290**: C262–70.

[113] Le Gars M, Descamps D, Roussel D, Saussereau E, Guillot L, et al. Neutrophil elastase degrades cystic fibrosis transmembrane conductance regulator via calpains and disables channel function in vitro and in vivo. Am J Respir Crit Care Med. 2013; **187**: 170–9.

[114] Twigg MS, Brockbank S, Lowry P, FitzGerald SP, Taggart C, et al. The role of serine proteases and antiproteases in the cystic fibrosis lung. Mediators Inflamm. 2015; **2015**: 293053.

[115] Padrines M, Wolf M, Walz A, Baggiolini M. Interleukin-8 processing by neutrophil elastase, cathepsin G and proteinase-3. FEBS Lett. 1994; **352**: 231–5.

[116] Gaggar A, Hector A, Bratcher PE, Mall MA, Griese M, et al. The role of matrix metalloproteases in cystic fibrosis lung disease. Eur Respir J. 2011; **38**: 721–7.

[117] Garratt LW, Sutanto EN, Ling KM, Looi K, Iosifidis T, et al. Matrix metalloproteinase activation by free neutrophil elastase contributes to bronchiectasis progression in early cystic fibrosis. Eur Respir J. 2015; **46**: 384–94.

[118] Amitani R, Wilson R, Rutman A, Read R, Ward C, et al. Effects of human neutrophil elastase and *Pseudomonas aeruginosa* proteinases on human respiratory epithelium. Am J Respir Cell Mol Biol. 1991; **4**: 26–32.

[119] Sommerhoff CP, Nadel JA, Basbaum CB, Caughey GH. Neutrophil elastase and cathepsin G stimulate secretion from cultured bovine airway gland serous cells. J Clin Invest. 1990; **85**: 682–9.

[120] Nakamura H, Yoshimura K, McElvaney NG, Crystal RG. Neutrophil elastase in respiratory epithelial lining fluid of individuals with cystic fibrosis induces interleukin-8 gene expression in a human bronchial epithelial cell line. J Clin Invest. 1992; **89**: 1478–84.

[121] Caldwell RA, Boucher RC, Stutts MJ. Neutrophil elastase activates near-silent epithelial Na+ channels and increases airway epithelial Na+ transport. Am J Physiol Lung Cell Mol Physiol. 2005; **288**: L813–9.

[122] Hamon Y, Jaillon S, Person C, Ginies JL, Garo E, et al. Proteolytic cleavage of the long pentraxin PTX3 in the airways of cystic fibrosis patients. Innate Immun. 2013; **19**: 611–22.

[123] Rubio F, Cooley J, Accurso FJ, Remold-O'Donnell E. Linkage of neutrophil serine proteases and decreased surfactant protein-A (SP-A) levels in inflammatory lung disease. Thorax. 2004; **59**: 318–23.

[124] Bratcher PE, Weathington NM, Nick HJ, Jackson PL, Snelgrove RJ, et al. MMP-9 cleaves SP-D and abrogates its innate immune functions in vitro. PLoS One. 2012; **7**: e41881.

[125] Berger M, Sorensen RU, Tosi MF, Dearborn DG, Doring G. Complement receptor expression on neutrophils at an inflammatory site, the Pseudomonas-infected lung in cystic fibrosis. J Clin Invest. 1989; **84**: 1302–13.

[126] Tosi MF, Zakem H, Berger M. Neutrophil elastase cleaves C3bi on opsonized Pseudomonas as well as CR1 on neutrophils to create a functionally important opsonin receptor mismatch. J Clin Invest. 1990; **86**: 300–8.

[127] van den Berg CW, Tambourgi DV, Clark HW, Hoong SJ, Spiller OB, et al. Mechanism of neutrophil dysfunction: neutrophil serine proteases cleave and inactivate the C5a receptor. J Immunol. 2014; **192**: 1787–95.

[128] Hartl D, Latzin P, Hordijk P, Marcos V, Rudolph C, et al. Cleavage of CXCR1 on neutrophils disables bacterial killing in cystic fibrosis lung disease. Nat Med. 2007; **13**: 1423–30.

[129] Vega-Carrascal I, Bergin DA, McElvaney OJ, McCarthy C, Banville N, et al. Galectin-9 signaling through TIM-3 is involved in neutrophil-mediated gram-negative bacterial killing: an effect abrogated within the cystic fibrosis lung. J Immunol. 2014; **192**: 2418–31.

[130] Farberman MM, Akers KT, Malone JP, Erdman-Gilmore P, Townsend RR, et al. Airway proteins involved in bacterial clearance susceptible to cathepsin G proteolysis. Eur Respir J. 2010; **35**: 410–7.

[131] Vandivier RW, Fadok VA, Ogden CA, Hoffmann PR, Brain JD, et al. Impaired clearance of apoptotic cells from cystic fibrosis airways. Chest. 2002; **121**: 89S.

[132] Valayer A, Brea D, Lajoie L, Avezard L, Combes-Soia L, et al. Neutrophils can disarm NK cell response through cleavage of NKp46. J Leukoc Biol. 2017; **101**: 253–9.

[133] Doring G, Frank F, boudier C, Herbert S, Fleischer B, et al. Cleavage of lymphocyte surface antigens CD2, CD4 and CD8 by polymorphonuclear leukocyte elastase and cathepsin G in patients with cystic fibrosis. J Immunol. 1995; **154**: 4842–50.

[134] Le-Barillec K, Si-Tahar M, Balloy V, Chignard M. Proteolysis of monocyte CD14 by human leukocyte elastase inhibits lipopolysaccharide-mediated cell activation. J Clin Invest. 1999; **103**: 1039–46.

[135] Reeves EP, McCarthy C, McElvaney OJ, Vijayan MS, White MM, et al. Inhaled hypertonic saline for cystic fibrosis: reviewing the potential evidence for modulation of neutrophil signalling and function. World J Crit Care Med. 2015; **4**: 179–91.

[136] Yang C, Chilvers M, Montgomery M, Nolan SJ. Dornase alfa for cystic fibrosis. Cochrane Database Syst Rev. 2016; **4**: CD001127.

[137] Borowitz D, Parad RB, Sharp JK, Sabadosa KA, Robinson KA, et al. Cystic Fibrosis Foundation practice guidelines for the management of infants with cystic fibrosis transmembrane conductance regulator-related metabolic syndrome during the first two years of life and beyond. J Pediatr. 2009; **155**: S106–16.

[138] Ramsey BW, Davies J, McElvaney NG, Tullis E, Bell SC, et al. A CFTR potentiator in patients with cystic fibrosis and the G551D mutation. N Engl J Med. 2011; **365**: 1663–72.

[139] Davies JC, Cunningham S, Harris WT, Lapey A, Regelmann WE, et al. Safety, pharmacokinetics, and pharmacodynamics of ivacaftor in patients aged 2–5 years with cystic fibrosis and a CFTR gating mutation (KIWI): an open-label, single-arm study. Lancet Respir Med. 2016; **4**: 107–15.

[140] Amaral MD. Novel personalized therapies for cystic fibrosis: treating the basic defect in all patients. J Intern Med. 2015; **277**: 155–66.

[141] Mayer-Hamblett N, Aitken ML, Accurso FJ, Kronmal RA, Konstan MW, et al. Association between pulmonary function and sputum biomarkers in cystic fibrosis. Am J Respir Crit Care Med. 2007; **175**: 822–8.

[142] Conese M, Castellani S, Lepore S, Palumbo O, Manca A, et al. Evaluation of genome-wide expression profiles of blood and sputum neutrophils in cystic fibrosis patients before and after antibiotic therapy. PLoS One. 2014; **9**: e104080.

[143] Bratcher PE, Rowe SM, Reeves G, Roberts T, Szul T, et al. Alterations in blood leukocytes of G551D-bearing cystic fibrosis patients undergoing treatment with ivacaftor. J Cyst Fibros. 2016; **15**: 67–73.

Section 3

Immunosuppressive Properties of Neutrophils

Chapter 7

Neutrophils Plasticity: The Regulatory Interface in Various Pathological Conditions

Suelen Martins Perobelli,
Triciana Gonçalves Silva and Adriana Bonomo

Additional information is available at the end of the chapter

http://dx.doi.org/10.5772/68130

Abstract

It is now known that neutrophils make up a population of complex cells with great plasticity, challenging the old view of neutrophil association with tissue damage and early phases of infection. Here, we discuss different contexts in which these cells can induce anti-inflammatory responses. Although distinct surface markers and cytokines profiles were shown, the most reliable characterization of suppressor neutrophil subtypes relies on their functional characteristics. One important example of inhibitory neutrophils generation comes from in vivo treatment with G-CSF, for 5 days, as for hematopoietic-stem-cell-transplantation (HSCT). In this case,donor blood is enriched in degranulated granulocytes harboring a functional regulatory phenotype, characterized by IL-10 production. These cells, when transferred together with HSCT, are able to reduce graft-versus-host-disease, being influenced by Treg cells and influencing them back. Importantly, this protection is long lasting and specific, keeping immunocompetence to other antigens. This regulation is paramount in HSCT, and represents a simple approach to be applied in humans. In summary, we discuss the interaction of neutrophils with other cell types and its consequence in immunomodulation. We believe these features confer an important bridge between innate and adaptive immune system, building a new knowledge for an underestimated cell type.

Keywords: regulatory neutrophils, neutrophils subtypes, T cell inhibition, Cytokines, G-CSF, GVHD

INTECH
open science | open minds

1. Introduction: Regulatory neutrophils and their profile

1.1. New technologies changing the concept of a short half-life

Besides the known features of neutrophils as fast migrating pro-inflammatory cells, the literature has shown that this is not a homogeneous population. In fact, several different subtypes of neutrophils have been well described regarding its characteristics and mechanisms of action. However, there are still some subtypes not so well understood.

The classical, and popular, concept of neutrophils says that they are the first cells to arrive and accumulate at the site of infections where they rapidly release several toxic molecules and undergo apoptosis [1]. In the meantime, they clear the infected area through phagocytosis or "neutrophils extracellular traps" (NETs) that occur when activated neutrophils release their uncondensed chromatin and granule contents. These molecules bind to pathogens causing death, contributing to fight against infections, and causing important tissue damage. Macrophages come over after this, clean up cell debris, and amplify the response [2, 3].

However, since different and modern techniques started to be accessible to research, some functions and concepts assigned to neutrophils have changed. The paradigm of the short half-life fell with the improvement of cellular techniques that enable better stains for different phenotypic markers or gene expressions. A variety of different neutrophils subtypes that are different in their phenotype, function, package of cytokines produced, degree of maturation, and site of action have been identified. So, a number of different types of neutrophils are being described including the ones with regulatory properties (hereafter referred as regulatory neutrophils—RN) that we will look closer in this chapter [4, 5].

How can these new findings interfere in the classic view of these cells?

Previously, a half-life of ~24 hours for human neutrophils and ~8 hours for murine neutrophils was believed. However, recently, using *in vivo* labeling techniques with ^2H_2O, a stable isotope, it was shown that human neutrophils in homeostatic conditions present an average 5.4 days of half-life [6]. The discrepancy with previous studies is believed to be due to *ex-vivo* manipulation and i.v. injection of neutrophils, which affects cells viability and *in vivo* distribution. Neutrophils longer half-life allows the conditions to develop phenotypic and functional alterations, including synthesis of a great number of cytokines, ability to recirculate and alter or influence other immune cells [7].

Neutrophils half-life can be dictated by several factors as inflammatory conditions, cytokines, cell interactions, PAMPS (pathogen-associated molecular pattern), and DAMPS (danger-associated molecular pattern), which might inhibit apoptosis and prolong the cell life span [8]. Then, this longer half-life associated with all sort of stimuli paves the way for new regulatory subtypes to emerge.

1.2. Neutrophil subtypes generated in specific conditions

The classical murine neutrophils can be identified by Ly6G$^+$ expression, while human neutrophils have to accomplish the expression of CD14, CD15, and CD16, always associated with a visual inspection that must identify a band or hypersegmented nucleus with a light pink cytoplasm, full of granules [4].

Although the existence of different neutrophils subtypes is currently accepted, the basis for their classification remains obscure. Distinct surface markers or new cytokines are common characteristics used to define neutrophils, but heterogeneity can also be explained by a stage of differential activation of neutrophil subpopulations [3, 7].

In some autoimmune diseases, such as systemic vasculitis associated (ASV) with anti-neutrophil cytoplasmic autoantibody or systemic lupus erythematous (SLE), circulating neutrophils display an increased expression of the specific surface marker, CD177. This is a molecule compartmentalized in secondary (specific) granule, that is co-expressed with its membrane ligand proteinase 3 (mPR3) in neutrophils from ASV patients. mPR3 is one of the main targets of ANCA autoantibodies, and, in this case, CD177 is important to mPR3 expression influencing the potential of neutrophils to be activated by ANCAs that usually target mPR3. However, levels of CD177 expression in patients and their influence on ANCA have not been defined as disease biomarkers yet, the $CD177^+$ neutrophils (NB1 in humans) represent indeed a new subset [9, 10].

Importantly in SLE, where the response is driven against nuclear antigens in various target organs such as the skin, kidney, and joints, neutrophils have been described as the source of DNA antigens due to its extravasation of nuclear content when forming NETs. Besides the $CD177^+$ NB1 neutrophils, low-density granulocytes (LDGs) are another subpopulation, which has been described in SLE. Specifically in this case, LDGs can assume a highly inflammatory profile, including the release of NETs, which amplifies disease physiopathology [11, 12]. The same LDG subtype was described in rheumatoid arthritis (RA). In RA, they show a low expression of TNFR, potentially affecting TNFi (inhibitor) treatment [13]. Beyond that, LDGs were also reported in mycobacterial infections being associated with disease severity [14]. This probably happens because it suppresses the immune response allowing mycobacterium growth. In severe asthma [15] and in interstitial lung disease in dermatomyositis [16], similar to what was described in autoimmune diseases like SLE and RA, the LDG acts worsening the pathologic condition.

The above features evidence the complex behavior of neutrophils requesting a lot more to be described about the plasticity of neutrophils in disease pathogenesis.

Apart from the uncommon profile of neutrophils in autoimmune diseases, we can highlight the phenotype of aged or senescent neutrophils. This particular subset expresses CXCR4 in high densities ($CXCR4^{hi}$). CXCR4 mediates cell retention in the bone marrow along with low expression of CD62L ($CD62L^{low}$). They express high CD11b and have hypersegmented nuclei [17]. Recently, it was described that ageing neutrophils are regulated by the microbiota in a toll-like receptor (TLR)-dependent way. The microbiota is the community of microorganisms that lives within the body and in harmony with it. The most studied group in this regard is bacteria from the human gastrointestinal (GI) tract that harbors an estimated $\sim 10^{14}$ individuals from about 1000 species in a single individual. Close to ~15,000 species of bacteria have already been identified from human GI samples [18]. These commensal bacteria can influence the immune system inducing a pro-inflammatory or a suppressor response, which depends on the bacteria quality and the milieu of activation. When the microbiota is depleted with the use of antibiotics, the number of aged neutrophils (that are highly activated cells) decreases, and the pathogenesis of sickle-cell disease or endotoxin-induced septic shock improves, showing that aged neutrophils have an important role in inflammatory diseases [19].

Another neutrophil subtype extremely relevant for immunology are the tumor-associated neutrophils (TAN), that are subdivided into type 1 (N1), with anti-tumor activity, and type 2 (N2), that fulfills a pro-tumor activity and will be discussed in the next subsection [20]. They have high relevance in the prognostic of some types of tumors, as colorectal [21], non-small cell lung [22], and breast where ratio of neutrophils/lymphocyte (NLR) is used as a toll to correlate with a better or poor prognostic [23].

Plasticity of TANs depends on many factors such as cytokines, chemokines, and adhesion molecules. These factors can be secreted by other immune cells or by the tumor itself [24]. The anti-inflammatory cytokine TGF-β has an important role in this scenario: in its presence, TANs can be directed to a pro-tumor N2 phenotype, and in its absence (using blocking antibodies) TANs are driven to an anti-tumor N1 phenotype [20]. On the other hand, these neutrophils can also interfere with the tumor microenvironment through the release of cytokines (TNF-α, IL-1β, IL-12), chemokines (CCL2, CCL3 and CCL5), reactive oxygen species (ROS), and growth factors, creating a diverse niche amplifying or down-regulating the inflammatory response [5, 25, 26]. Phenotypically, the N1 type presents a hypersegmentated nuclei with high expression of FAS, ICAM, and TNF-α production, making them able to activate TCD8+ lymphocytes, helping to eliminate the tumor cells [20].

These ambiguous characteristics evidence how the plasticity of neutrophils can impact in health and in pathological conditions. Until now, we covered how neutrophils can assume different subtypes and contribute to a pro-inflammatory milieu, amplifying the immune responses in autoimmune diseases as well in highly activated conditions, as the aged neutrophils in inflammatory infections. In tumor setting, the ratio neutrophil/lymphocyte can even predict the patient prognostic highlighting the importance of neutrophils in disease outcome.

In Section 1.3, we describe the profile of RN, the conditions in which they were described their mechanism of action, and the possibility to manipulate them for therapeutic usage.

1.3. Regulatory neutrophil phenotypes

As stated above, nowadays, the literature accepts that neutrophils can assume different subtypes. It is important to point here that the term "regulatory" or "suppressor" indicates the capacity of these cells to induce an anti-inflammatory response, either by interacting directly with other cells or by secreting molecules that induce polarization of other cell types.

The classification of RN subtypes is still unclear. The most reliable characterization of the suppressor neutrophil subtypes remains being their functional characteristics. Although there are some markers, such as $CD62L^{low}/CD11b^{low}$ highly associated with suppressor phenotypes and others such as CD244, CD115, CD11c, CD32, CD35, CD45, and CD66b, which can be up-regulated, there is no consensus for a specific combination of markers for suppressor neutrophils. Their phenotype heterogeneity is probably because they are modulated according to individual conditions [3, 4]. So, in this section, we discuss the literature on the different subtypes (or phenotypes) of RN.

Among the subtypes described, we can highlight the granulocytic myeloid-derived suppressor cells (G-MDSCs), which are an important sub-population of circulating neutrophils [27]. MDSCs are a heterogeneous population of immature and mature cells, of myeloid origin, first described in tumor-bearing mice and comprise two groups of cells identified regarding their morphology and phenotype. Monocyte-MDSCs (M-MDSCs) are $CD11b^{+}Ly6C^{high}Ly6G^{-}$ and have a typical monocyte morphology, and cells $CD11b^{+}Ly6C^{low}Ly6G^{+}$ with typical granulocytic morphology are G-MDSC [28, 29]. The G-MDSC phenotype is characterized mainly by large amounts of ROS expression and low amounts of nitric oxide synthase (NOS). The opposite is true for the M-MDSC phenotype that acts mainly expressing arginase-1 (Arg1) and NOS. MDSCs can inhibit T cell responses in many ways. After being generated as a consequence of intense inflammatory environment in the presence of factors like GM-CSF (granulocyte-macrophage colony stimulating factor), G-CSF (granulocyte colony stimulating factor), VEGF, IL-6, MDSCs are recruited to the site of the primary tumor and secondary lymphoid organs (lymph nodes, spleen) by chemokines such as CCL2, CXCL12, and CXCL5 [30]. Upon arrival in the specific site, they can modify the microenvironment by secreting NOS, ARG, and/or ROS.

Although described as harmful in autoimmune diseases, it is also known that mouse and human LDGs are a heterogeneous population composed of mature and immature neutrophils with suppressive capacity. Neutrophils are classified as LDG or low-density neutrophils (LDNs) and high-density granulocytes (HDNs) depending on their density. In general, LDG or LDN cells co-purify with PBMC at the low-density layer in a ficoll gradient, rather than with the high-density layer, which is the usual for the classic neutrophils [31, 32].

It was shown in a tumor model that LDN comprises at least two different populations: one with a segmented nucleus (mature) and another with banded or ring-shaped nucleus (immature) that resembles the G-MDSC phenotype. Both can be generated from HDN in a TGF-β-dependent way. In this case, a new nomenclature was suggested to circulating mature neutrophils. The HDN that are pro-inflammatory with anti-tumor profile would be called Nc1 and its counterpart mature LDN, which shows a pro-tumor activity would be Nc2. The Nc2 has reduced expression of inflammatory molecules and inhibit $TCD8^{+}$ proliferation *in vitro* evidencing more than one type of RN [32].

During pregnancy, where immunosuppressive state is required to allow implantation and growth of the fetus, an important population of LDG producing arginase-1 was identified in PBMC and placentae of pregnant women and in the cord blood. Besides, these neutrophils were described as cells that released specific granules (once they increase expression of CD66b), and the azurophilic granules, where arginase-1 is stored (once CD63 is expressed). These phenotypical markers associated with others mean that these cells have been activated and are degranulated. Presence of arginase-1 collaborates to impair T cell responses once the L-arginine deprivation induced by release of arginase contributes to T cell hyporesponsiveness and immune privilege at the materno-fetal interface [33, 34].

In HIV infection, LDGs act to inhibit the immune system, worsening the condition. PBMCs from HIV-infected patients are rich in high arginase LDGs, suggesting that they are activated neutrophils that had degranulated [35].

Some years ago, our group observed that LDG was increased in the peripheral blood of G-CSF-treated donors of peripheral blood stem cells. These cells were capable to inhibit T cells IL-4 and IFN-γ production in a hydrogen peroxide (H_2O_2)-dependent way [36]. In a murine model of graft versus host disease (GVHD), the main limitation of stem cell transplantation, LDGs prevented 100% mortality [31]. These cells were better characterized recently [37] and will be described at the end of this chapter.

On the other hand, in infection with methicillin-resistant *Staphylococcus aureus* strain, three different subtypes of mouse neutrophils with different susceptibilities to infection have been described. Besides the normal PMN-N (polymorphonuclear neutrophils), there are at least two distinct PMN subtypes (PMN-I and PMN-II). The suppressor subtype (PMN-II) can express TLR2/TLR4/TLR7/TLR9 and has low levels of MPO (myeloperoxidases). PMN-II is involved with the generation of alternatively activated macrophages (M2), through IL-10- and CCL2-dependent mechanisms. These M2 macrophages have anti-inflammatory properties and induce a Th2 response [38], modulating the adaptive immune response at the expense of neutrophils.

Regarding cytokines production, RN IL-10$^+$ producing cells have been described. The IL-10 is an important cytokine, which can be produced by many different cell types, as B cells, mast cells, eosinophils, macrophages, DCs, and a large number of T cell subtypes that act regulating the synthesis of pro-inflammatory chemokines and cytokines, such as IL-1, IL-6, TNF-α, as well as nitric oxide (NO), collagenase, and gelatinase [3, 39, 40].

In murine models, several studies have shown that neutrophils produce IL-10 in response to a variety of infections, such as *S. aureus* [38], *Candida albicans* [40], *Trypanssoma cruzi* [41], and in inflammatory conditions, such as post-burn [42] and after G-CSF treatment [37]. However, these data are still a matter of conflict in the literature since just a few studies show the same phenotype in humans [43–45] and others were incapable to reproduce it [46, 47].

These differences in IL-10 production between mouse and human neutrophils may result from different factors, such as culture conditions, contaminating cells, or post-transcriptional regulation of IL-10 gene expression [47, 48].

Moreover, the cytokine IL-22 has also been described as being produced by neutrophils, besides being produced by many different cells, including Th17, Th22, NK cells, Tγδ, and ILC (innate-like lymphocytes). RN IL-22$^+$ is mainly important for intestinal barrier maintenance exerting a local modulation and keeping the integrity of the intestinal mucosa, generating a protective response against certain extracellular pathogenic bacteria [49, 50]. IL-22 has the ability to synergize with other cytokines to induce gene expression of antimicrobial peptides, chemokines, matrix metalloproteinase, cytokines, and epithelial acute phase proteins in the skin, liver, lung, and intestine [51, 52]. Of note, it was described that neutrophil-producing IL-22 has an important role in intestinal protection in a model of colitis. The adoptive transfer of IL-22-producing neutrophils to IL-22-deficient animals was protective for dextran-induced colitis inducing the release of antimicrobial peptides RegIIIβ and S100A8 by colonic cells, protecting the intestinal barrier from microbes and helping the resolution of disease [53].

At last, as stated before, in tumor settings, neutrophils can assume ambiguous features being supportive or inhibiting the tumor growth. We described above the TAN-N1 pro-inflammatory neutrophils, protecting from tumor, but it is also important to highlight the TAN-N2 neutrophils that are suppressive and, in this case, harmful for the patient. N2 TANs are tumor resident neutrophils that influence the establishment, development, and spread of cancers. They can be generated in a TGF-β milieu and also by G-CSF produced by tumor cells, among others [20]. Under G-CSF stimuli, neutrophils are generated and expand, creating a pro-tumorigenic niche, being able to favor metastatic microenviroment [54]. TAN-N2 cells express arginase, contributing to inhibition of T cell responses. They release chemokines such as CCL2 and CCL5 that favor the recruitment of other cell types, including regulatory T cells (Tregs). Also, they can produce oncostatin-M that works promoting angiogenesis and neovascularization favoring tumor growth [20, 55, 56]. Depletion of neutrophils from tumor-bearing mice shows an increase in $TCD8^+$ cells, supporting the concept that N2 acts in a suppressive way being an RN [20]. As stated above, the ratio between lymphocytes and neutrophils (NLR) is used to predict the patient prognosis in cancer patients. In breast tumors, a high NLR is associated with a poor prognostic and a shorter overall survival [57].

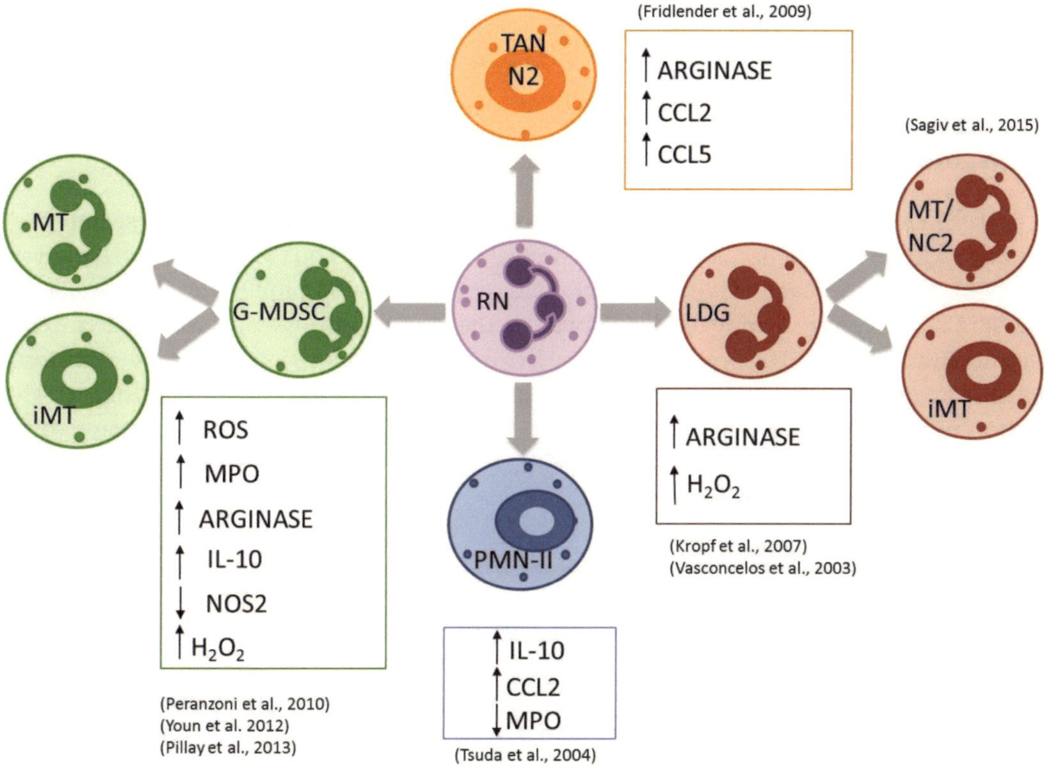

Figure 1. Illustration of the most well-described regulatory neutrophils (RN) subtypes and their main mechanisms of action. TAN-N2 (Tumor associated neutrophil type 2); G-MDSC (Granulocytic myeloid derived suppressor cell); PMN-II (Polymorphonuclear type II); LDG (low-density granulocyte); NC2 (circulating neutrophils type 2); MT (mature); iMT (immature).

Despite those RN that share some similarities regarding their mechanism of action based on arginase production, H_2O_2, Treg induction by IL-10 secretion, and M2 generation, there are still some differences among the cell types that prevent them from being placed in the same general group of RN. Many authors have been trying to establish a nomenclature to these RN; however, new subsets keep being described as well as new features which make this a hard task and fill the literature with different names, many times for the same described cell. Some of the subsets are well defined as MDSC, like high-density mature, low-density mature or immature, as can be seen in **Figure 1**. In this regard, these cells can express different markers, be sensitive to diverse stimuli, and influence different cell types showing important consequences in amplification of suppressive immune response. The crosstalk of neutrophils with other cell types and the maintenance of the suppressor "tonus" will be explored in more details in Section 2 (**Figure 1**).

2. Changes in the immune response under neutrophils influence

As mentioned earlier, neutrophils are recruited to different tissues after injury or infection and, in this sites, encounter resident and/or recruited leukocytes, which promote interactions that influence each other mutually. Under neutrophil influence, other cell types acquire regulatory properties worsening or improving the host condition. On the other hand, neutrophils can suffer influences that polarize them to a suppressor phenotype.

2.1. Neutrophil influence in macrophage polarization

In *Nippostrongylus brasiliensis* infection, neutrophils acquire a N2 phenotype that secrete high amount of IL-13 that in turn is essential to provide helper functions to promote alternatively activated M2 macrophage polarization with long-lived profile. The M2 macrophages mediate parasitic larval damage during recall responses in the lung and are essential to nematode damage and clearance [58]. The presence of these M2 macrophages also impairs host antibacterial resistance against sepsis. In thermally injured mice, PMN-II displays an immunosuppressive phenotype with production of CCL2 and IL-10. These induce macrophages conversion to M2 favoring *Enterococcus faecalis* translocation [59]. The same mechanism was also described in humans with severe burn injuries [60].

2.2. NK, NKT, and ILCs suppression by neutrophils

Neutrophils are also able to inhibit NK cell activity. *In vitro* co-culture assay demonstrated that in the presence of neutrophils and G-MDSCs, there was a significant decrease in NKp30 expression that led to a reduced NK cell cytotoxicity against *Aspergillus fumigatus*. Moreover, activation markers CD69 and CD137 expression and secretion of the effector molecule IFN-γ were also decreased in NK cells incubated with neutrophils or G-MDSCs before the infection with *A. fumigatus* [61]. In vaccinia virus infection, the G-MDSC subset was responsible for the NK function and proliferation inhibition mediated by ROS [62]. A crucial role of primary tumor-mobilized neutrophils and NK crosstalk in the establishment of lung pre-metastatic niches was described. In this case, they are able to inhibit NK cell-mediated clearance of metastatic cells and simultaneously promoting intraluminal survival and extravasation at the metastatic site. *In vitro* functional assay of lung NK cells obtained from tumor-bearing mice showed that these cells were significantly less responsive to the NKG2D or NKp46, NK-activating receptors (measured by expression of CD107 and IFN-γ) than the naïve mice [63]. Reciprocally, human NK cells (resting or activated by IL-12) were able to induce neutrophil apoptosis dependent on cell-cell contact and caspases, which overcome the antiapoptotic effect of GM-CSF. Involvement of the activating NK cell receptor NKp46 and the Fas pathway was observed in this process [64]. This regulatory effect of NK cells on neutrophils was also observed in the DSS-induced colitis model. However, in this model, NK cells significantly lowered the percentage of apoptotic neutrophils in co-cultured assay. The regulatory effect is dependent on down-regulation of the inflammatory neutrophil functions (decrease in IL-6 and increase in IL-10 production) and is largely dependent on direct NK cell-neutrophil contact, via their inhibitory receptor NKG2A [65].

Mouse and human invariant NKT (iNKT) cells were also inhibited by contact with live neutrophils. iNKT cells from mice with acute inflammatory neutrophilia (as in peritonitis) display decrease in T-bx21 and GATA3 expression and diminished cytokine production compared with those from control mice. *In vitro* assay demonstrated that cell-cell contact between iNKT and neutrophils is required for the inhibitory effect and that this encounter impairs the cytotoxicity capacity of iNKT cells [66].

The relationship between neutrophils and innate lymphoid cells (ILC3) was shown in human decidua during pregnancy. The ILCs are important effectors of innate immunity present in small amounts in lymphoid tissues and enriched at barrier surfaces, such as the skin, lung, intestine, and mucosal-associated lymphoid tissues. Characterized by the absence of recombination activating gene (RAG)-dependent rearranged antigen receptors, lack of myeloid cell and dendritic cell phenotypical markers and lymphoid morphology, ILCs undergo neither clonal selection nor expansion when stimulated. These cells reflect the phenotypes and functions of T lymphocytes and NK cells. There are at least three subtypes of ILCs, which are named ILC1, ILC2, and ILC3. They represent the innate counterparts of $CD4^+$ Th1, Th2, and Th17, respectively [67–69]. It has been observed that the numbers of Natural Cytotoxic Receptors positive ILC 3 (NCR^+ ILC3) infiltrating decidual tissues positively correlate with those of infiltrating neutrophils. Neutrophils are present in human decidua during the first trimester of normal pregnancy but not in spontaneous miscarriages decidua. *In vitro* assays show that decidual NCR^+ ILC3 release CXCL8 and GM-CSF and can induce neutrophil migration and survival, respectively. Moreover, NCR^+ ILC3-derived GM-CSF induces expression of HB-EGF and of IL1rα in neutrophils that have anti-inflammatory activity and helps to mediate trophoblast invasion, pointing out a possible role of these cells in the early phases of pregnancy [70].

2.3. Dendritic cells on the neutrophils target

The crosstalk between neutrophils and dendritic cells (DC) can be deleterious for DC functions in *Leishmania major* infection. When neutrophils from ear dermis of C57BL/6-infected mice were cultured with bone marrow-derived dendritic cells, they were engulfed by the DC. These DCs show a significant reduction in expression of MHC class II, CD40, and CD86, as well as an inhibited capacity to stimulate T CD8+ lymphocytes proliferation and IFN-γ production. These effects were mediated by the tyrosine kinase receptor "Mer" expressed on DCs [71].

The immunosuppressive effect of apoptotic and necrotic neutrophils was also observed in humans' DC. *In vitro,* DC phagocytes apoptotic/necrotic neutrophils and display up-regulation of CD83 and MHC II. However, a decrease of important molecules that stimulate T lymphocytes as CD40, CD80, and CD86 was observed showing that apoptotic/necrotic neutrophils are able to induce a suppressor immune response through DC modulation [72].

DCs infected with *Mycobacterium bovis* (BCG) produced high levels of CXCL1 and CXCL2 that attract neutrophils. In this process, the close contact mediated by CD11b between DCs and neutrophils induces the production of large amounts of the immunosuppressive cytokine IL-10 via MyD88 and Syk pathways in neutrophils. These IL-10+ neutrophils specifically shut down IL-17A production by Th17 cells. This mechanism could break IL-17A production and avoid exacerbated neutrophil recruitment modulating inflammation [73].

MPO is an enzyme found in neutrophils azurophilic granules and is important for intracellular pathogen killing. It was demonstrated that MPO is deposited by neutrophils in lymph nodes, where it interacts with DCs (by catalytic activity through various ROS and DC Mac-1). In this way, MPO is involved in DC changes during the induction of adaptive immunity. DC display reduced activation, defect in uptake/processing antigens, and inhibited migration to LNs by reduced expression of CCR7, leading to reduced adaptive immune response [74].

Neutrophil elastase is a serine proteinase stored in neutrophils azurophilic granules that can damage endothelial cells and cleave endothelial cell-associated adhesion molecules. As MPO, elastase shows modulating effect on DCs. In presence of elastase, immature DC increases the expression of TGFβ-1 and decreases the IL-6, as well their ability to allostimulate T cells. Elastase-treated dendritic cells not only inhibit the proliferation of allogeneic T cells but also increase TGF-β1 expression inducing the differentiation higher number of CD4+ Foxp3+ Treg cells in MLR cultures. Together, these data suggest mechanisms by which tolerogenic DCs generated by neutrophils elastase exposure contribute to immune regulation [75, 76].

2.4. Neutrophils and B cells crosstalk

During *S. aureus* infection, neutrophils infiltrate the draining lymph nodes, occupying the medulla and interfollicular areas. These cells form transient and long-lived interactions with B lymphocytes and plasma cells inducing a decrease in B cell IgM production in a TGF- β1 dependent manner [77].

Site-specific splenic neutrophils function as professional helper cells for marginal zone B cells, specialized area in T cell-independent responses to circulating antigen, leading to the generation of affinity-matured antibodies. Neutrophils colonize the marginal zone of the spleen after postnatal mucosal colonization by microbiota. In the spleen, these neutrophils interact with local macrophages that produce IL-10, splenic sinusoidal endothelial cells, that in response to the microbial TLR ligands secrete IL-10 and neutrophil-attracting chemokines, and other STAT3-activating stromal factors, which induce modification of neutrophils phenotype, acquiring a "B cell-helper phenotype." These neutrophils B-cell helper (NBH) are divided into two subpopulation according to their molecule profile expression. NBH1 cells had intermediate expression of CD15 and CD16 and NBH2 cells had low expression of CD15 and CD16. Despite their morphological and ultrastructural similarity to NBH2 cells, NBH1 cells were more activated than NBH2 cells, as they had higher expression of CD27, CD40L, CD86, CD95, and HLA-II but lower expression of CD24. Relative to genes expression (mRNA abundance) compared with "conventional neutrophils," NBH1 and NBH2 cells had more abundant mRNA immunoregulatory molecules, such as IL-10, IL-10 receptor, arginase-1, RALDH1, iNOS, IDO, SOCS1, progranulin, and SLPI, suggesting a skew toward a regulatory profile. In fact, these neutrophils could suppress CD4 proliferation in a contact-independent way. Thus, NBH cells could function as professional MZ B cell helper cells and may suppress T cells to induce immunoglobulin responses in a T-independent manner. These NBH cells were specially characterized by their higher expression of CD40L and surface BAFF and released high amounts of BAFF, APRIL and IL-21, crucial molecules for the B cell functions [78].

2.5. T cell activities under neutrophils control

Finally, we will describe one of the most important crosstalk of neutrophils, which can have long-term consequences: interactions with T cells. The mechanisms involved in the T cells suppression by neutrophils can be achieved by depletion of essential amino acids from the microenvironment, such as L-arginine, generation of ROS, or through cell-cell contact. Neutrophils produce large amounts of arginase-1 that are stocked in gelatinase granules. Release of arginase-1 requires cellular activation and degranulation of gelatinase and azurophilic granules. Arginase is an enzyme that metabolizes L-arginine into L-ornithine and urea. L-arginine is crucial to T cell proliferation, in the absence of it T lymphocytes are arrested in the G0–G1 phase of the cell cycle. Also, in the absence of L-arginine, expression of TCRζ (CD3 zeta chain) is down-regulated and cofilin dephosphorylation is impaired affecting F-actin remodeling, which is essential for T cell effector function [79–82].

Another important mediator of neutrophil-T cell inter-talk is the ROS, which are membrane-permeable and act on neighboring cells. Peroxide (H_2O_2) can suppress lymphocyte proliferation by decreasing NF-κB activation, down-regulating TCRζ and oxidating cofilin. H_2O_2 has a short half-life and is degraded by many endogenous anti-oxidants. Thus, a close contact between neutrophils and T lymphocyte is required for the suppressor effect. The cell-to-cell contact is mediated by expression of the integrin CD11b/CD18 in neutrophil [4, 83, 84].

The cell-cell contact mediated immunosuppression on T cells can be through a PD-L1-PD1 pathway. PD1 is a negative co-stimulatory receptor expressed primarily on activated T cells. Its main role is to limit the effector functions of T cells during inflammatory response. When engaged by one of its ligands, PD1 inhibits kinases, which reduces cytokine production and suppresses T cell proliferation [85, 86]. In volunteers who participated in a human endotoxemia clinical trial, submitted to LPS inoculums, was observed an accumulation of suppressive neutrophils ($CD16^{hi}$ $CD62L^{lo}$) that exhibit an increased expression of PD-L1 gene and membrane-bound molecule, which was attributed a exposure and stimulation of these cells with IFN-γ and to a lesser extend IFN-α or IFN-β. These IFN-γ-treated neutrophils were able to inhibit proliferation of polyclonal-activated T cells in PD-L1 and cell-cell contact-dependent mechanism [87]. The same phenomenon was observed in murine model of sepsis [88].

In HIV-infected patients, neutrophils play an unappreciated role contributing to the chronic state of immunosuppression leading to opportunistic infection. Low-density neutrophils (which display the same phenotype of G-MDSC) from the peripheral blood of HIV-1 viremic patients express high level of PD-L1. The PD-L1 expression on neutrophils was regulated by the interaction of these cells with inactivated HIV-1 virions, IFN-α, and TLR-7 and TLR-8 ligands. These neutrophils suppress T cell function via PD-L1/PD-1 interaction and production of ROS [89]. The same suppressive function was also observed in *Burkholderia pseudomallei* infected neutrophils, that up-regulated expression of PD-L1 and was able to inhibit $CD4^+$ T cell proliferation and IFN-γ production in response to polyclonal activators, mediated by the PD-L1/PD-1 pathway [90].

Thus, as can be seen in **Figure 2**, the subtypes of RN as well as their diverse interactions with other cell types perform an amplification of the immune response that may help or hinder the host. In Section 3, we describe in details the mechanism of action of an important regulatory neutrophil subtype in GVHD control (**Figure 2**).

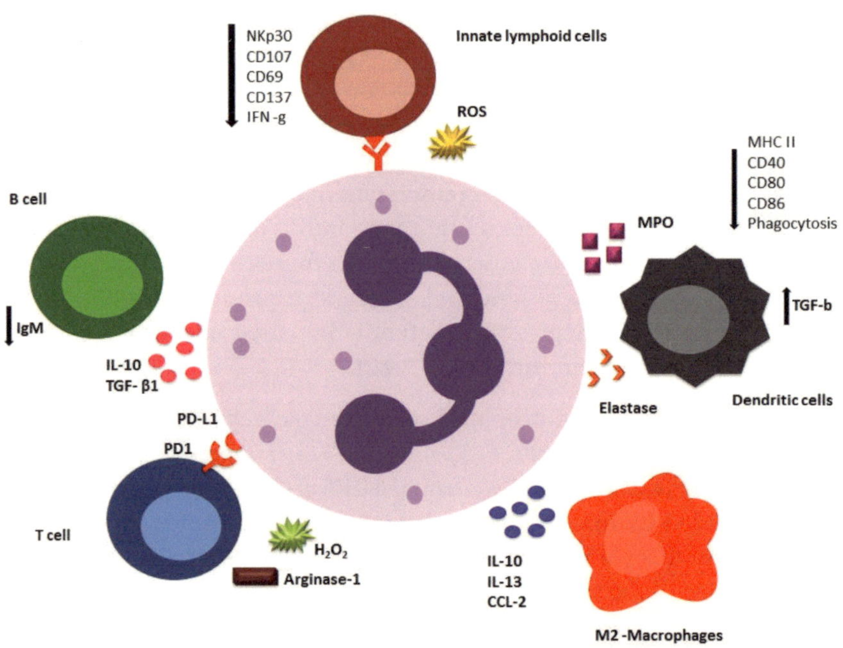

Figure 2. Regulatory neutrophils act on immune cells playing immunosuppressive role. Neutrophil MPO and elastase induce decrease in uptake/antigens processing by DC, inhibit migration to the lymph nodes, and their ability to stimulate T cells are impaired. Also, elastase induces TGF-β1 production by DC. Moreover, the uptake of apoptotic neutrophils down-modulates expression of MHCII, CD40, CD80, and CD86. The secretion cytokines IL-10, IL-13, and chemokine CCL-2 are implicated in the ability of neutrophils to induce changes in macrophages phenotypes to the "M2" anti-inflammatory kind. The immunossuppression of neutrophils over T cells is mediated by the production of ROS, ARG-1, and co-inhibitory molecule PD-L1. Moreover, neutrophils secret IL-10 that exert suppression of T cells functions. TGB-β1 secretion by neutrophils directly influences humoral response by decreasing IgM production. Splenic neutrophils display a particular profile, which produces high amounts of soluble factors essential to the B cells maintenance and also express IL-10. ROS production by neutrophils and cell-cell contact between ILC and neutrophils decreases cytotoxicity, reduces ILC responsiveness to activator receptor, and down-modulates expression of NKp30, CD69, CD137, CD107, and of IFN-γ.

http://dx.doi.org/10.5772/68130

3. Role of regulatory neutrophils in GVHD protection

GVHD is characterized by a robust adaptive immune response caused by donor T cells (present in the incoming graft) after hematopoietic stem cells transplantation (HSCT), a frequent treatment for hematopoietic disorders, and leukemia. In order to be transplanted, the receptor patient undergoes a conditioning regimen that consists of radio/chemotherapy that eliminates the disease and creates the niche for the new incoming bone marrow cells. However, the conditioning regimen also damages the epithelial cells of the patient, mainly the gastrointestinal mucosa, with barrier breakdown and microbiota extravasation. In this case, when donor cells arrive, they find an inflammatory milieu and the T cells are activated by host antigen-presenting cells (APCs) in an inflammatory context and migrate to organs such as the gut, skin, liver, and lungs. The result is the development of GVHD, which has high morbidity and mortality rates, and is the most important limitation of HSCT [91, 92]. Although it is well known that GVHD is mediated and dependent on T cells, elimination of T cells from the graft does eliminate the GVHD. However, it brings other undesired consequences as the lack of anti-leukemia response and deficient hematopoiesis with bone marrow failure [92].

As mentioned before, LDGs have been found in PBMC of stem cell donors treated with G-CSF. These cells were described to be able to inhibit IFN-γ and IL-4 production by T cells in a H_2O_2-dependent way [36]. In the mouse model for GVHD, the same suppressor phenotype was found, and these LDGs were able to inhibit experimental GVHD [31].

Recently, we extended these results showing, among other things, that Ly6G$^+$ RN mediates disease inhibition. In a mouse model of hematopoietic stem cell transplantation (HSCT), after G-CSF treatment, donor spleen cells are enriched in neutrophils (from ~2 to ~20%) and, as related in the literature by others, Treg cells were also increased [93, 94]. However, depleting Treg cells from the graft does not alter the GVHD outcome while depleting neutrophils Ly6G$^+$ causes a huge detriment to clinical scores and survival rates. In terms of GVHD, it is important to point that protection was long-lasting and specific, keeping the immunocompetence to reject the skin grafts from third-party mice and rejecting the leukemic cells, keeping the GVL effect. These results show that neutrophils instruct T cells toward a specific tolerant state [37].

So, looking closer to RN, it is important to note that treatment with G-CSF increased the Ly6G$^+$Ly6C$^-$ population but not the Ly6G$^-$Ly6C$^+$ or Ly6G$^+$Ly6C$^+$ population consistent with the enrichment of neutrophils but not macrophages or MDSC [95, 96]. The RN has a reduction in the expression of some surface molecules, such as MHC-II, CD62L, and co-stimulatory (CD80, CD86, CD40), increased phagocytic capacity and produce large amounts of H_2O_2 molecules. Under stimuli in culture, they produce low IFN-γ, TNF-α, IL-17F, IL-2, IL-12 while increasing IL-22 and the suppressor cytokine IL-10. Also, they have low arginase-1 expression and high NOS, associated with low levels of MPO, which justifies the high amount of H_2O_2. Altogether, these features encompass a different subtype of suppressor neutrophils.

Confirming that IL-10 production is particularly important to GVHD suppression, transference of a G-CSF-induced neutrophil from IL-10-deficient mice in a HSCT context, abolished GVHD protection showing high mortality rates and poor clinical scores. This evidences that IL-10$^+$ neutrophils are the agents of protection [37].

Nevertheless, the long-lasting and specific protection cannot be explained only by neutrophils suppression as it lasts for several months and the half-life of neutrophils does not exceed 6 days. When analyzing the amount of Treg cells, in spleen and mesenteric lymph nodes (mLN) of the hosts, it was found that 4 days after HSCT, Tregs were increased on mLN but not on spleens. Moreover, 25 days after HSCT, both spleen and MLN show Treg increase, suggesting a systemic increase in Treg. In this way, when Treg cells are depleted early after the transplantation, the GVHD protection is abolished, showing Treg induction within the host right after transplantation. These specific suppressor effects are compatible with the antigen-specific suppression previously observed with Treg cells [97, 98]. The ability of neutrophils to suppress T cell activation is reinforced by the fact that Tregs are less sensitive than conventional T cells to H_2O_2 suppression [99].

Indeed, it's known that G-CSF treatment increases the number of Treg cells in the donor, and that these cells produce IL-10 [93]. Treg cells stimulated with LPS are able to induce IL-10 and TGFβ-producing neutrophils. It means that Treg cells have anti-inflammatory properties that influence other cells, including neutrophils, which upon contact with LPS-stimulated Tregs, may prevent the induction of the Th17 profile [100] (**Figure 3**).

Given these various functions of the $Ly6G^+$ $IL\text{-}10^+$ neutrophils described herein, at least three possibilities, which may act together, can be suggested to explain the specific suppression by RN in GVHD model.

At first, peroxide production can act by inhibiting T cell activation because its production is carried out with L-arginine consumption and because it acts by inhibiting TCRζ chain phosphorylation. Second, the high phagocytic capacity may contribute to the clearance of translocated gut bacteria after the conditioning regimen. The diminished bacterial load and translocation will contribute to diminished activation of allogeneic T cells leading to a mild GVHD. Third, Tregs generated in the donor after G-CSF treatment influence the generation and modulation of spleen neutrophils to an $IL\text{-}10^+$-producing suppressor subtype, which expresses low levels of MHC II and co-stimulation (as can be seen in **Figure 4**). After HSCT, when in contact with T cells, neutrophils with low levels of co-stimulatory molecules associated with high secretion of IL-10 favor the generation of Treg cells within the host that suppresses GVHD and maintains other functions of the immune system while maintaining immunocompetence and the GVL effect (**Figure 4**).

In addition to this, we believe that the high phagocytic capacity found in these neutrophils, coupled with the high production of H_2O_2, is related to the limitation of bacterial extravasation that occurs as a result of the barrier breaking [101]. It was recently described that neutrophils can colonize intestinal tissues 3 days after transplantation, so the $Ly6G^+$ cell, besides polarizing T cells, could maintain the intestinal integrity [102]. In fact, it has already been described that G-CSF decreases the effects of intestinal barrier breakage showing low levels of endotoxin in the blood and lower numbers of translocated bacteria observed in the spleen, liver, and mesenteric lymph nodes compared to those not treated with G-CSF [103]. Bacterial elimination is of utmost importance for the control of GVHD, so much that it has been described that germ-free animals develop an attenuated and very late form of GVHD [104]. Besides this, in our view, in this early phase after HSCT neutrophils polarize T cells in

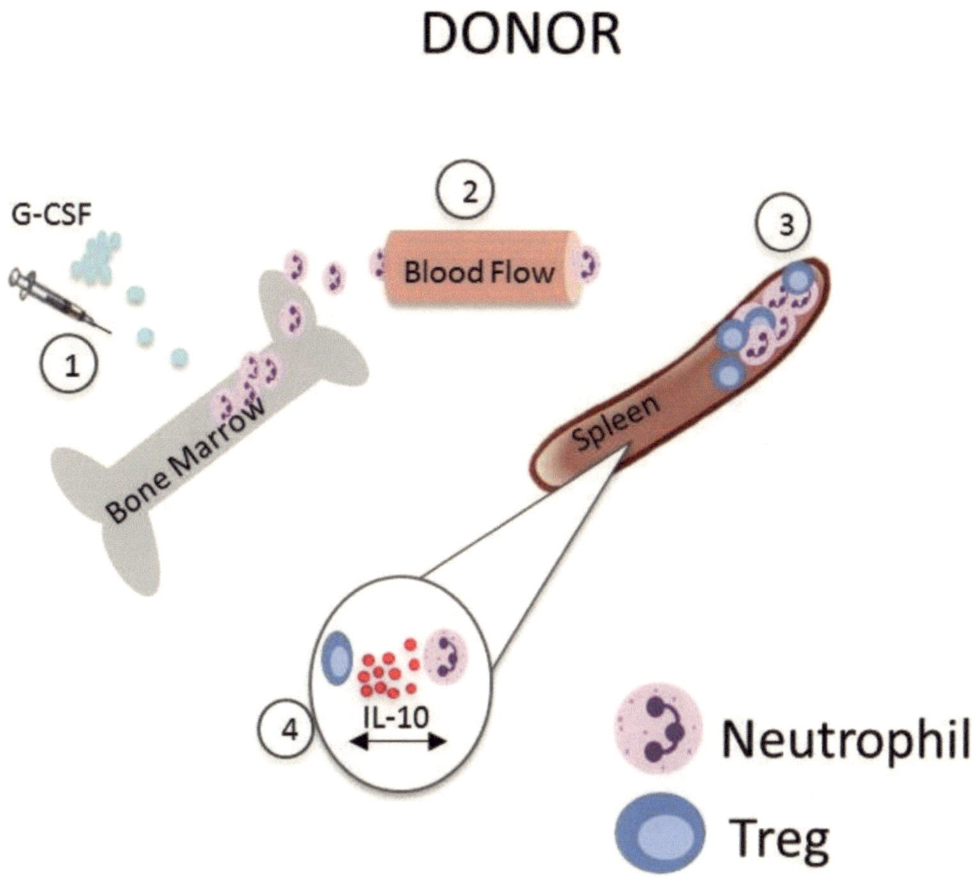

Figure 3. Regulatory neutrophils IL10+ neutrophils generation. (1) G-CSF treatment of HSCT donors mobilizes neutrophils from the bone marrow to the periphery. (2) and (3) Neutrophils migrate to spleen where they found Treg cells also G-CSF stimulated. (4) In the spleen, neutrophils and T cells undergo mutual influence and polarize each other to a regulatory phenotype.

the mLN towards a regulatory phenotype, and these regulatory cells spread to GVHD target organs, as we suggest in **Figure 4**.

As we can conclude, the initial idea that neutrophils act only by responding rapidly to inflammatory stimuli and subsequently enter apoptosis causing tissue damage has been modified by the finding that activated neutrophils can perform many other functions. Studies in this regard challenge the classical view of neutrophils as fully differentiated cells and raise the question that these cells may exhibit extraordinary plasticity. In GVHD, prevention strategies that spare the recipient or that decrease tissue damage are of extreme importance [100]. In this case, the generation of a new subtype of neutrophils, capable of inhibiting GVHD maintaining the immunological competence, is paramount for the control of the disease and represents a simple approach to be applied in humans.

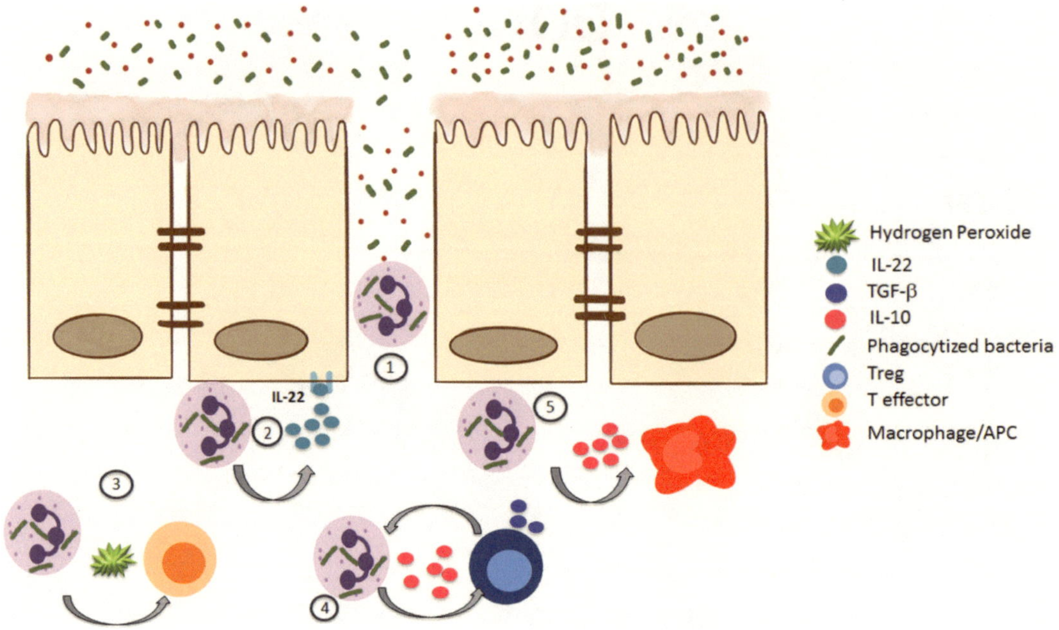

Figure 4. Potential role of regulatory neutrophils in GVHD onset. (1) After HSCT, regulatory neutrophils limit the bacterial translocation from the intestinal barrier breakdown, once they have high phagocytic capacity. (2) Production of the cytokine IL-22 contributes to epithelial healing. (3) High levels of hydrogen peroxide inhibit T effect or functions protecting the host from clonal expansion of alloreactive T cells. (4) The IL10 derived from neutrophils, polarize host Tregs and this last produces IL-10 and TGF-β comprising a mutual cycle. (5) Alternative macrophage (M2) differentiation can be influenced by the regulatory milieu.

4. Final considerations

In mouse model, treatment with G-CSF generates in the HSCT donors an increase of Treg cells, which may be responsible for the generation of suppressor neutrophils. When transferred to the HSCT receptors, these neutrophils are able to suppress the GVHD by reducing the clinical and histopathological signs of the disease. On the other hand, these protected individuals retain the anti-leukemia effect, which is important to prevent relapses, and reject allogeneic skin grafts, showing that the protection of GVHD is due to a specific suppression and not a systemic immunosuppression of the recipient, which claims for a T cell function.

The type of neutrophil generated after G-CSF treatment is obviously different from the classical neutrophil, known as inflammatory. Although activated and mature, they express low levels of MHC-II and co-stimulatory molecules, low levels of MPO, and are degranulated. On the other hand, they are producers of the suppressive cytokine IL-10 and also show an increase in IL-4 and IL-22. Together, these characteristics make this cell a potential suppressor, since several mechanisms able to modulate T cells are present.

We believe that after transfer to the recipient, these neutrophils (which have a longer half-life, as recently reported in the literature) rapidly colonize the sites activated by the conditioning regimen. It is known that in 3 days there is neutrophil colonization in mLN. Although reports in the literature associate this early neutrophil colonization with the increased damage caused by GVHD, this neutrophil is of a distinct subtype, generated after treatment with G-CSF. Thus, in these activated sites, neutrophils can act to control local inflammation, generating a regulatory environment, favoring the generation of new Treg cells that amplify the specific protection observed in our study.

We conclude that neutrophils function goes beyond the microbicidal function. The classical view is too narrow to explain the many features acquired by these cells. Many different and complex subtypes of regulatory neutrophils have been recently described. Although their characterization is not precise, regulatory neutrophils can be grouped together based on their functional profile. Also, the interaction between these neutrophils and other cell types, such as the ones described here (macrophages, NK, NKT, ILC, DC, B and T cells), potentiate the regulatory response in different conditions. So, the regulatory neutrophils confer an important bridge between innate and adaptive immune system in many different conditions, building a new role for an underestimated cell.

Author details

Suelen Martins Perobelli, Triciana Gonçalves Silva and Adriana Bonomo*

*Address all correspondence to: acbonomo@gmail.com

Laboratory of Thymus Research, Oswaldo Cruz Institute, Oswaldo Cruz Foundation, Rio de Janeiro, Brazil

References

[1] de Oliveira S, Rosowski EE, Huttenlocher A (2016): Neutrophil migration in infection and wound repair: going forward in reverse. Nat Rev Immunol 16, 378–91

[2] Mitsios A, Arampatzioglou A, Arelaki S, Mitroulis I, Ritis K (2016): NETopathies? Unraveling the dark side of old diseases through neutrophils. Front Immunol 7, 678

[3] Perobelli SM, Galvani RG, Gonçalves-Silva T, Xavier CR, Nóbrega A, Bonomo A (2015): Plasticity of neutrophils reveals modulatory capacity. Braz J Med Biol Res 48, 665–75

[4] Pillay J, Tak T, Kamp VM, Koenderman L (2013): Immune suppression by neutrophils and granulocytic myeloid-derived suppressor cells: similarities and differences. Cell Mol Life Sci 70, 3813–27

[5] Mantovani A, Cassatella MA, Costantini C, Jaillon S (2011): Neutrophils in the activation and regulation of innate and adaptive immunity. Nat Rev Immunol 11, 519–31

[6] Pillay J, den Braber I, Vrisekoop N, Kwast LM, de Boer RJ, Borghans JA, Tesselaar K, Koenderman L (2010): In vivo labeling with ^2H_2O reveals a human neutrophil lifespan of 5.4 days. Blood 116, 625–7

[7] Silvestre-Roig C, Hidalgo A, Soehnlein O (2016): Neutrophil heterogeneity: implications for homeostasis and pathogenesis. Blood 127, 2173–81

[8] Geering B, Stoeckle C, Conus S, Simon HU (2013): Living and dying for inflammation: neutrophils, eosinophils, basophils. Trends Immunol 34, 398–409

[9] Hu N, Westra J, Huitema MG, Bijl M, Brouwer E, Stegeman CA, Heeringa P, Limburg PC, Kallenberg CG (2009): Coexpression of CD177 and membrane proteinase 3 on neutrophils in antineutrophil cytoplasmic autoantibody-associated systemic vasculitis: anti-proteinase 3-mediated neutrophil activation is independent of the role of CD177-expressing neutrophils. Arthritis Rheum 60, 1548–57

[10] Amulic B, Cazalet C, Hayes GL, Metzler KD, Zychlinsky A (2012): Neutrophil function: from mechanisms to disease. Annu Rev Immunol 30, 459–89

[11] Midgley A, Beresford MW (2016): Increased expression of low density granulocytes in juvenile-onset systemic lupus erythematosus patients correlates with disease activity. Lupus 25, 407–11

[12] Carmona-Rivera C, Kaplan MJ (2013): Low-density granulocytes: a distinct class of neutrophils in systemic autoimmunity. Semin Immunopathol 35, 455–63

[13] Wright HL, Makki FA, Moots RJ, Edwards SW (2017): Low-density granulocytes: functionally distinct, immature neutrophils in rheumatoid arthritis with altered properties and defective TNF signalling. J Leukoc Biol 101, 599–611

[14] Deng Y, Ye J, Luo Q, Huang Z, Peng Y, Xiong G, Guo Y, Jiang H, Li J (2016): Low-density granulocytes are elevated in mycobacterial infection and associated with the severity of tuberculosis. PLoS One 11, e0153567

[15] Fu J, Tobin MC, Thomas LL (2014): Neutrophil-like low-density granulocytes are elevated in patients with moderate to severe persistent asthma. Ann Allergy Asthma Immunol 113, 635–640.e2

[16] Zhang S, Shen H, Shu X, Peng Q, Wang G (2017): Abnormally increased low-density granulocytes in peripheral blood mononuclear cells are associated with interstitial lung disease in dermatomyositis. Mod Rheumatol 27, 122–9

[17] Casanova-Acebes M, Pitaval C, Weiss LA, Nombela-Arrieta C, Chèvre R, A-González N, Kunisaki Y, Zhang D, van Rooijen N, Silberstein LE, Weber C, Nagasawa T, Frenette PS, Castrillo A, Hidalgo A (2013): Rhythmic modulation of the hematopoietic niche through neutrophil clearance. Cell 153, 1025–35

[18] Shono Y et al. (2016): Increased GVHD-related mortality with broad-spectrum antibiotic use after allogeneic hematopoietic stem cell transplantation in human patients and mice. Sci Transl Med 8, 339ra71

[19] Zhang D, Chen G, Manwani D, Mortha A, Xu C, Faith JJ, Burk RD, Kunisaki Y, Jang JE, Scheiermann C, Merad M, Frenette PS (2015): Neutrophil ageing is regulated by the microbiome. Nature 525, 528–32

[20] Fridlender ZG, Sun J, Kim S, Kapoor V, Cheng G, Ling L, Worthen GS, Albelda SM (2009): Polarization of tumor-associated neutrophil phenotype by TGF-beta: "N1" versus "N2" TAN. Cancer Cell 16, 183–94

[21] Walsh SR, Cook EJ, Goulder F, Justin TA, Keeling NJ (2005): Neutrophil-lymphocyte ratio as a prognostic factor in colorectal cancer. J Surg Oncol 91, 181–4

[22] Sarraf KM, Belcher E, Raevsky E, Nicholson AG, Goldstraw P, Lim E (2009): Neutrophil/lymphocyte ratio and its association with survival after complete resection in non-small cell lung cancer. J Thorac Cardiovasc Surg 137, 425–8

[23] Chen J, Deng Q, Pan Y, He B, Ying H, Sun H, Liu X, Wang S (2015): Prognostic value of neutrophil-to-lymphocyte ratio in breast cancer. FEBS Open Bio 5, 502–7

[24] Kobayashi Y (2008): The role of chemokines in neutrophil biology. Front Biosci 13, 2400–7

[25] Gabrilovich DI, Nagaraj S (2009): Myeloid-derived suppressor cells as regulators of the immune system. Nat Rev Immunol 9, 162–74

[26] Gregory AD, Houghton AM (2011): Tumor-associated neutrophils: new targets for cancer therapy. Cancer Res 71, 2411–6

[27] Mishalian I, Granot Z, Fridlender ZG (2017): The diversity of circulating neutrophils in cancer. Immunobiology 222, 82–8

[28] Youn JI, Collazo M, Shalova IN, Biswas SK, Gabrilovich DI (2012): Characterization of the nature of granulocytic myeloid-derived suppressor cells in tumor-bearing mice. J Leukoc Biol 91, 167–81

[29] Peranzoni E, Zilio S, Marigo I, Dolcetti L, Zanovello P, Mandruzzato S, Bronte V (2010): Myeloid-derived suppressor cell heterogeneity and subset definition. Curr Opin Immunol 22, 238–44

[30] Heim CE, Vidlak D, Kielian T (2015): Interleukin-10 production by myeloid-derived suppressor cells contributes to bacterial persistence during *Staphylococcus aureus* orthopedic biofilm infection. J Leukoc Biol 98, 1003–13

[31] Vasconcelos ZF, Dos Santos BM, Farache J, Palmeira TS, Areal RB, Cunha JM, Barcinski MA, Bonomo A (2006): G-CSF-treated granulocytes inhibit acute graft-versus-host disease. Blood 107, 2192–9

[32] Sagiv JY, Michaeli J, Assi S, Mishalian I, Kisos H, Levy L, Damti P, Lumbroso D, Polyansky L, Sionov RV, Ariel A, Hovav AH, Henke E, Fridlender ZG, Granot Z (2015): Phenotypic diversity and plasticity in circulating neutrophil subpopulations in cancer. Cell Rep 10, 562–73

[33] Kropf P, Baud D, Marshall SE, Munder M, Mosley A, Fuentes JM, Bangham CR, Taylor GP, Herath S, Choi BS, Soler G, Teoh T, Modolell M, Müller I (2007): Arginase activity mediates reversible T cell hyporesponsiveness in human pregnancy. Eur J Immunol 37, 935–45

[34] Ssemaganda A, Kindinger L, Bergin P, Nielsen L, Mpendo J, Ssetaala A, Kiwanuka N, Munder M, Teoh TG, Kropf P, Müller I (2014): Characterization of neutrophil subsets in healthy human pregnancies. PLoS One 9, e85696

[35] Cloke TE, Garvey L, Choi BS, Abebe T, Hailu A, Hancock M, Kadolsky U, Bangham CR, Munder M, Müller I, Taylor GP, Kropf P (2010): Increased level of arginase activity correlates with disease severity in HIV-seropositive patients. J Infect Dis 202, 374–85

[36] Vasconcelos ZF, Santos BM, Costa ES, Lima M, Tabak DG, Bouzas LF, Azevedo WM, Barcinski MA, Bonomo A (2003): T-lymphocyte function from peripheral blood stem-cell donors is inhibited by activated granulocytes. Cytotherapy 5, 336–45

[37] Perobelli SM, Mercadante AC, Galvani RG, Gonçalves-Silva T, Alves AP, Pereira-Neves A, Benchimol M, Nóbrega A, Bonomo A (2016): G-CSF-induced suppressor IL-10+ neutrophils promote regulatory T cells that inhibit graft-versus-host disease in a long-lasting and specific way. J Immunol 197, 3725–3734

[38] Tsuda Y, Takahashi H, Kobayashi M, Hanafusa T, Herndon DN, Suzuki F (2004): Three different neutrophil subsets exhibited in mice with different susceptibilities to infection by methicillin-resistant *Staphylococcus aureus*. Immunity 21, 215–26

[39] Zhang Q, Chen B, Yan F, Guo J, Zhu X, Ma S, Yang W (2014): Interleukin-10 inhibits bone resorption: a potential therapeutic strategy in periodontitis and other bone loss diseases. Biomed Res Int 2014, 284836

[40] Mencacci A, Cenci E, Spaccapelo R, Tonnetti L, del Sero G, d'Ostiani CF, Bistoni F, Romani L (1996): Neutrophils producing interleukin-10 antagonize the effect of interleukin-12 in mice with candidiasis. Ann N Y Acad Sci 795, 394–6

[41] Tosello Boari J, Amezcua Vesely MC, Bermejo DA, Ramello MC, Montes CL, Cejas H, Gruppi A, Acosta Rodríguez EV (2012): IL-17RA signaling reduces inflammation and mortality during *Trypanosoma cruzi* infection by recruiting suppressive IL-10-producing neutrophils. PLoS Pathog 8, e1002658

[42] Noel G, Wang Q, Schwemberger S, Hanson C, Giacalone N, Haar L, Ogle CK (2011): Neutrophils, not monocyte/macrophages, are the major splenic source of postburn IL-10. Shock 36, 149–55

[43] Lewkowicz N, Mycko MP, Przygodzka P, Ćwiklińska H, Cichalewska M, Matysiak M, Selmaj K, Lewkowicz P (2016): Induction of human IL-10-producing neutrophils by LPS-stimulated Treg cells and IL-10. Mucosal Immunol 9, 364–78

[44] Balderramas HA, Penitenti M, Rodrigues DR, Bachiega TF, Fernandes RK, Ikoma MR, Dias-Melicio LA, Oliveira SL, Soares Â (2014): Human neutrophils produce IL-12, IL-10, PGE2 and LTB4 in response to *Paracoccidioides brasiliensis*. Involvement of TLR2, mannose receptor and dectin-1. Cytokine 67, 36–43

[45] De Santo C, Arscott R, Booth S, Karydis I, Jones M, Asher R, Salio M, Middleton M, Cerundolo V (2010): Invariant NKT cells modulate the suppressive activity of IL-10-secreting neutrophils differentiated with serum amyloid A. Nat Immunol 11, 1039–46

[46] Davey MS, Tamassia N, Rossato M, Bazzoni F, Calzetti F, Bruderek K, Sironi M, Zimmer L, Bottazzi B, Mantovani A, Brandau S, Moser B, Eberl M, Cassatella MA (2011): Failure to detect production of IL-10 by activated human neutrophils. Nat Immunol 12, 1017–8; author reply 1018–20

[47] Tamassia N, Zimmermann M, Castellucci M, Ostuni R, Bruderek K, Schilling B, Brandau S, Bazzoni F, Natoli G, Cassatella MA (2013): Cutting edge: an inactive chromatin configuration at the IL-10 locus in human neutrophils. J Immunol 190, 1921–5

[48] Powell MJ, Thompson SA, Tone Y, Waldmann H, Tone M (2000): Posttranscriptional regulation of IL-10 gene expression through sequences in the 3′-untranslated region. J Immunol 165, 292–6

[49] Marchesi F, Martin AP, Thirunarayanan N, Devany E, Mayer L, Grisotto MG, Furtado GC, Lira SA (2009): CXCL13 expression in the gut promotes accumulation of IL-22-producing lymphoid tissue-inducer cells, and formation of isolated lymphoid follicles. Mucosal Immunol 2, 486–94

[50] Sanos SL, Bui VL, Mortha A, Oberle K, Heners C, Johner C, Diefenbach A (2009): RORgammat and commensal microflora are required for the differentiation of mucosal interleukin 22-producing NKp46+ cells. Nat Immunol 10, 83–91

[51] Jenq RR et al. (2012): Regulation of intestinal inflammation by microbiota following allogeneic bone marrow transplantation. J Exp Med 209, 903–11

[52] Ouyang W, Valdez P (2008): IL-22 in mucosal immunity. Mucosal Immunol 1, 335–8

[53] Zindl CL, Lai JF, Lee YK, Maynard CL, Harbour SN, Ouyang W, Chaplin DD, Weaver CT (2013): IL-22-producing neutrophils contribute to antimicrobial defense and restitution of colonic epithelial integrity during colitis. Proc Natl Acad Sci USA 110, 12768–73

[54] Kowanetz M et al. (2010): Granulocyte-colony stimulating factor promotes lung metastasis through mobilization of Ly6G+Ly6C+ granulocytes. Proc Natl Acad Sci USA 107, 21248–55

[55] Aldinucci D, Colombatti A (2014): The inflammatory chemokine CCL5 and cancer progression. Mediators Inflamm 2014, 292376

[56] Queen MM, Ryan RE, Holzer RG, Keller-Peck CR, Jorcyk CL (2005): Breast cancer cells stimulate neutrophils to produce oncostatin M: potential implications for tumor progression. Cancer Res 65, 8896–904

[57] Faria SS, Fernandes PC, Silva MJ, Lima VC, Fontes W, Freitas-Junior R, Eterovic AK, Forget P (2016): The neutrophil-to-lymphocyte ratio: a narrative review. Ecancermedicalscience 10, 702

[58] Chen F, Wu W, Millman A, Craft JF, Chen E, Patel N, Boucher JL, Urban JF, Kim CC, Gause WC (2014): Neutrophils prime a long-lived effector macrophage phenotype that mediates accelerated helminth expulsion. Nat Immunol 15, 938–46

[59] Tsuda Y, Shigematsu K, Kobayashi M, Herndon DN, Suzuki F (2008): Role of polymorphonuclear neutrophils on infectious complications stemming from *Enterococcus faecalis* oral infection in thermally injured mice. J Immunol 180, 4133–8

[60] Yoshida T, Tsuda Y, Takeuchi D, Kobayashi M, Pollard RB, Suzuki F (2006): Glycyrrhizin inhibits neutrophil-associated generation of alternatively activated macrophages. Cytokine 33, 317–22

[61] Mueller-Leisse J, Brueggemann S, Bouzani M, Schmitt AL, Einsele H, Loeffler J (2015): Polymorphonuclear neutrophils and granulocytic myeloid-derived suppressor cells inhibit natural killer cell activity toward *Aspergillus fumigatus*. Med Mycol 53, 622–9

[62] Fortin C, Huang X, Yang Y (2012): NK cell response to vaccinia virus is regulated by myeloid-derived suppressor cells. J Immunol 189, 1843–9

[63] Spiegel A, Brooks MW, Houshyar S, Reinhardt F, Ardolino M, Fessler E, Chen MB, Krall JA, DeCock J, Zervantonakis IK, Iannello A, Iwamoto Y, Cortez-Retamozo V, Kamm RD, Pittet MJ, Raulet DH, Weinberg RA (2016): Neutrophils suppress intraluminal NK cell-mediated tumor cell clearance and enhance extravasation of disseminated carcinoma cells. Cancer Discov 6, 630–49

[64] Thorén FB, Riise RE, Ousbäck J, Della Chiesa M, Alsterholm M, Marcenaro E, Pesce S, Prato C, Cantoni C, Bylund J, Moretta L, Moretta A (2012): Human NK Cells induce neutrophil apoptosis via an NKp46- and Fas-dependent mechanism. J Immunol 188, 1668–74

[65] Hall LJ, Murphy CT, Quinlan A, Hurley G, Shanahan F, Nally K, Melgar S (2013): Natural killer cells protect mice from DSS-induced colitis by regulating neutrophil function via the NKG2A receptor. Mucosal Immunol 6, 1016–26

[66] Wingender G, Hiss M, Engel I, Peukert K, Ley K, Haller H, Kronenberg M, von Vietinghoff S (2012): Neutrophilic granulocytes modulate invariant NKT cell function in mice and humans. J Immunol 188, 3000–8

[67] Sonnenberg GF, Artis D (2015): Innate lymphoid cells in the initiation, regulation and resolution of inflammation. Nat Med 21, 698–708

[68] Artis D, Spits H (2015): The biology of innate lymphoid cells. Nature 517, 293–301

[69] Spits H, Artis D, Colonna M, Diefenbach A, Di Santo JP, Eberl G, Koyasu S, Locksley RM, McKenzie AN, Mebius RE, Powrie F, Vivier E (2013): Innate lymphoid cells--a proposal for uniform nomenclature. Nat Rev Immunol 13, 145–9

[70] Croxatto D, Micheletti A, Montaldo E, Orecchia P, Loiacono F, Canegallo F, Calzetti F, Fulcheri E, Munari E, Zamò A, Venturini PL, Moretta L, Cassatella MA, Mingari MC, Vacca P (2016): Group 3 innate lymphoid cells regulate neutrophil migration and function in human decidua. Mucosal Immunol 9, 1372–83

[71] Ribeiro-Gomes FL, Romano A, Lee S, Roffê E, Peters NC, Debrabant A, Sacks D (2015): Apoptotic cell clearance of *Leishmania major*-infected neutrophils by dendritic cells inhibits CD8⁺ T-cell priming in vitro by Mer tyrosine kinase-dependent signaling. Cell Death Dis 6, e2018

[72] Clayton AR, Prue RL, Harper L, Drayson MT, Savage CO (2003): Dendritic cell uptake of human apoptotic and necrotic neutrophils inhibits CD40, CD80, and CD86 expression and reduces allogeneic T cell responses: relevance to systemic vasculitis. Arthritis Rheum 48, 2362–74

[73] Doz E, Lombard R, Carreras F, Buzoni-Gatel D, Winter N (2013): Mycobacteria-infected dendritic cells attract neutrophils that produce IL-10 and specifically shut down Th17 CD4 T cells through their IL-10 receptor. J Immunol 191, 3818–26

[74] Odobasic D, Kitching AR, Yang Y, O'Sullivan KM, Muljadi RC, Edgtton KL, Tan DS, Summers SA, Morand EF, Holdsworth SR (2013): Neutrophil myeloperoxidase regulates T-cell-driven tissue inflammation in mice by inhibiting dendritic cell function. Blood 121, 4195–204

[75] Maffia PC, Zittermann SE, Scimone ML, Tateosian N, Amiano N, Guerrieri D, Lutzky V, Rosso D, Romeo HE, Garcia VE, Issekutz AC, Chuluyan HE (2007): Neutrophil elastase converts human immature dendritic cells into transforming growth factor-beta1-secreting cells and reduces allostimulatory ability. Am J Pathol 171, 928–37

[76] Tateosian NL, Reiteri RM, Amiano NO, Costa MJ, Villalonga X, Guerrieri D, Maffía PC (2011): Neutrophil elastase treated dendritic cells promote the generation of CD4(+) FOXP3(+) regulatory T cells in vitro. Cell Immunol 269, 128–34

[77] Kamenyeva O, Boularan C, Kabat J, Cheung GY, Cicala C, Yeh AJ, Chan JL, Periasamy S, Otto M, Kehrl JH (2015): Neutrophil recruitment to lymph nodes limits local humoral response to *Staphylococcus aureus*. PLoS Pathog 11, e1004827

[78] Puga I et al. (2011): B cell-helper neutrophils stimulate the diversification and production of immunoglobulin in the marginal zone of the spleen. Nat Immunol 13, 170–80

[79] Rodriguez PC, Quiceno DG, Ochoa AC (2007): L-arginine availability regulates T-lymphocyte cell-cycle progression. Blood 109, 1568–73

[80] Rodriguez PC, Zea AH, Culotta KS, Zabaleta J, Ochoa JB, Ochoa AC (2002): Regulation of T cell receptor CD3zeta chain expression by L-arginine. J Biol Chem 277, 21123–9

[81] Feldmeyer N, Wabnitz G, Leicht S, Luckner-Minden C, Schiller M, Franz T, Conradi R, Kropf P, Müller I, Ho AD, Samstag Y, Munder M (2012): Arginine deficiency leads to impaired cofilin dephosphorylation in activated human T lymphocytes. Int Immunol 24, 303–13

[82] Rotondo R, Bertolotto M, Barisione G, Astigiano S, Mandruzzato S, Ottonello L, Dallegri F, Bronte V, Ferrini S, Barbieri O (2011): Exocytosis of azurophil and arginase 1-containing granules by activated polymorphonuclear neutrophils is required to inhibit T lymphocyte proliferation. J Leukoc Biol 89, 721–7

[83] Malmberg KJ, Arulampalam V, Ichihara F, Petersson M, Seki K, Andersson T, Lenkei R, Masucci G, Pettersson S, Kiessling R (2001): Inhibition of activated/memory (CD45RO(+)) T cells by oxidative stress associated with block of NF-kappaB activation. J Immunol 167, 2595–601

[84] Schmielau J, Finn OJ (2001): Activated granulocytes and granulocyte-derived hydrogen peroxide are the underlying mechanism of suppression of t-cell function in advanced cancer patients. Cancer Res 61, 4756–60

[85] Sharpe AH, Freeman GJ (2002): The B7-CD28 superfamily. Nat Rev Immunol 2, 116–26

[86] Pardoll DM (2012): The blockade of immune checkpoints in cancer immunotherapy. Nat Rev Cancer 12, 252–64

[87] de Kleijn S, Langereis JD, Leentjens J, Kox M, Netea MG, Koenderman L, Ferwerda G, Pickkers P, Hermans PW (2013): IFN-γ-stimulated neutrophils suppress lymphocyte proliferation through expression of PD-L1. PLoS One 8, e72249

[88] Wang JF, Li JB, Zhao YJ, Yi WJ, Bian JJ, Wan XJ, Zhu KM, Deng XM (2015): Up-regulation of programmed cell death 1 ligand 1 on neutrophils may be involved in sepsis-induced immunosuppression: an animal study and a prospective case-control study. Anesthesiology 122, 852–63

[89] Bowers NL, Helton ES, Huijbregts RP, Goepfert PA, Heath SL, Hel Z (2014): Immune suppression by neutrophils in HIV-1 infection: role of PD-L1/PD-1 pathway. PLoS Pathog 10, e1003993

[90] Buddhisa S, Rinchai D, Ato M, Bancroft GJ, Lertmemongkolchai G (2015): Programmed death ligand 1 on *Burkholderia pseudomallei*-infected human polymorphonuclear neutrophils impairs T cell functions. J Immunol 194, 4413–21

[91] Shlomchik WD, Lee SJ, Couriel D, Pavletic SZ (2007): Transplantation's greatest challenges: advances in chronic graft-versus-host disease. Biol Blood Marrow Transplant 13, 2–10

[92] Heidegger S, van den Brink MR, Haas T, Poeck H (2014): The role of pattern-recognition receptors in graft-versus-host disease and graft-versus-leukemia after allogeneic stem cell transplantation. Front Immunol 5, 337

[93] Morris ES, MacDonald KP, Rowe V, Johnson DH, Banovic T, Clouston AD, Hill GR (2004): Donor treatment with pegylated G-CSF augments the generation of IL-10-producing regulatory T cells and promotes transplantation tolerance. Blood 103, 3573–81

[94] Reisner Y, Aversa F, Martelli MF (2015): Haploidentical hematopoietic stem cell transplantation: state of art. Bone Marrow Transplant 50 Suppl 2, S1–5

[95] Ostrand-Rosenberg S (2008): Immune surveillance: a balance between protumor and antitumor immunity. Curr Opin Genet Dev 18, 11–8

[96] Höchst B, Mikulec J, Baccega T, Metzger C, Welz M, Peusquens J, Tacke F, Knolle P, Kurts C, Diehl L, Ludwig-Portugall I (2015): Differential induction of Ly6G and Ly6C positive myeloid derived suppressor cells in chronic kidney and liver inflammation and fibrosis. PLoS One 10, e0119662

[97] Mercadante AC, Perobelli SM, Alves AP, Gonçalves-Silva T, Mello W, Gomes-Santos AC, Miyoshi A, Azevedo V, Faria AM, Bonomo A (2014): Oral combined therapy with

probiotics and alloantigen induces B cell-dependent long-lasting specific tolerance. J Immunol 192, 1928–37

[98] Gomez JC, Yamada M, Martin JR, Dang H, Brickey WJ, Bergmeier W, Dinauer MC, Doerschuk CM (2015): Mechanisms of interferon-γ production by neutrophils and its function during *Streptococcus pneumoniae* pneumonia. Am J Respir Cell Mol Biol 52, 349–64

[99] Mougiakakos D, Johansson CC, Kiessling R (2009): Naturally occurring regulatory T cells show reduced sensitivity toward oxidative stress-induced cell death. Blood 113, 3542–5

[100] Lewkowicz N, Klink M, Mycko MP, Lewkowicz P (2013): Neutrophil--CD4+CD25+ T regulatory cell interactions: a possible new mechanism of infectious tolerance. Immunobiology 218, 455–64

[101] Holler E, Landfried K, Meier J, Hausmann M, Rogler G (2010): The role of bacteria and pattern recognition receptors in GVHD. Int J Inflam 2010, 814326

[102] Schwab L et al. (2014): Neutrophil granulocytes recruited upon translocation of intestinal bacteria enhance graft-versus-host disease via tissue damage. Nat Med 20, 648–54

[103] Zhang C, Xu YG, Duan XN, Liu YH, Zhao JX, Xu L, Ye JM (2011): Role of granulocyte colony-stimulating factor in paclitaxel-induced intestinal barrier breakdown and bacterial translocation in rats. Chin Med J (Engl) 124, 1870–5

[104] van Bekkum DW, Roodenburg J, Heidt PJ, van der Waaij D (1974): Mitigation of secondary disease of allogeneic mouse radiation chimeras by modification of the intestinal microflora. J Natl Cancer Inst 52, 401–4